Exchanges for All Occasions

Meeting the Challenge of Diabetes

Marion J. Franz, R.D., M.S.

Wellness
And
Nutrition
Library

Diabetes Center, Inc.

Editor: Donna Hoel
Indexing: Audrey DeLaMarte
Typesetting: Associated Litho
Printing: Associated Litho

©1983, revised 1987
International Diabetes Center

Published by Diabetes Center, Inc.
P.O. Box 739
Wayzata, Minnesota 55391

Printed in the United States of America
10   9   8   7   6   5   4   3   2   1

PREFACE

Much has happened in the area of nutrition and diabetes management since the original **Exchanges for All Occasions** was written in 1983. It has been an exciting time!

Exchange Lists for Meal Planning, the guidebook to nutrition management published by the American Diabetes Association and the American Dietetic Association, was revised in 1986 to reflect nutrition and food composition data as we understand it now. This 1987 version of **Exchanges for All Occasions** expands on that information.

This new edition has been completely revised. Nutritional recommendations and principles for persons with diabetes have been re-examined. It has become clearer how important nutrition is in the overall management of diabetes. However, at the same time, our new information reinforces the idea that the nutritional recommendations for persons with diabetes are similar to those for all Americans!

The basic principles of diabetes management remain the same—balancing food, insulin and exercise. More information about food can help persons with diabetes meet this lifetime challenge. Attention to meal planning is essential if the goal of maintaining normal blood glucose levels is to be achieved.

Nutritional recommendations for individuals with diabetes can benefit all family members. The 1985 **Dietary Guidelines for Americans** has this advice for choosing and preparing healthy foods: Eat a variety of foods; maintain ideal weight; avoid too much fat, saturated fat, and cholesterol; eat foods with adequate starch and fiber; avoid too much sugar and salt; and if you drink alcohol, do so in moderation. Sound familiar? This is very similar to what is recommended for persons with diabetes.

This book has been written to help those with diabetes add variety, flexibility and interest to their meal plans and to help health professionals with nutritional counseling.

It is my hope this book will allow individuals to enjoy their meals and social life while carefully following meal plans.

A very special thanks to Donna Hoel for her help in the editing and production of this book. Thanks also to the wonderful and professionally skilled dietitians on the staff of the International Diabetes Center—Gay Castle, Nancy Cooper, Broatch Haig, Arlene Monk, Gretchen Morin, Diane Reader—for their ideas, help and support. And finally, a thank you to Donnell D. Etzwiler, M.D., Judy Joynes, R.N., Bill Henry and the I.D.C. staff for their continued support and encouragement. They are all grand!

Marion J. Franz
Director of Nutrition
International Diabetes Center

TABLE OF CONTENTS

Part IV   GUIDELINES FOR FOOD PURCHASING AND PREPARATION

TABLES

SAMPLE MENUS

Part I

EXPANDED EXCHANGE LISTS

Chapter One
FROM STARVATION
TO FIBER

Many changes have occurred in the management of diabetes since the discovery of insulin in 1921. And, of course, researchers are still finding ways to help individuals manage diabetes better. Nutrition is one area where ideas have changed drastically over the years.

Before the discovery and use of insulin in 1921, individuals were treated with "starvation diets." *Starvation Treatment of Diabetes* by Hill and Eckman in 1917 offers an example of how starvation diets were used:

> **Details of treatment.** *Forty-eight hours after admission to the hospital the patient is kept on ordinary diet to determine severity of his diabetes. Then he is starved, and no food allowed, some whiskey and black coffee, whiskey is given in the coffee: 1 ounce of whiskey every two hours, from 7 A.M. to 7 P.M. This furnishes roughly about 800 calories. The whiskey is not an essential part of the treatment; it merely furnishes a few calories and keeps the patient more comfortable while he is being starved.*

Alcohol was used because the body can use it as a source of energy without the help of insulin. Carbohydrate, protein, and fat — the nutrients that supply energy in everyday foods — all require insulin in order to supply energy or for them to be stored for future energy needs.

Diets for people with diabetes changed drastically after the discovery of insulin. Leonard Thompson, the first patient to receive insulin therapy in 1921, was placed on an excessively high fat diet for more than 12 years in the belief that it would improve his condition.

Diets that contain large amounts of fat are now known to contribute to the development of coronary heart disease. In addition, persons who have diabetes are at a very high risk for the development of coronary heart disease. Mr. Thompson's diet reportedly included 50 grams of protein (200 calories), 160 grams of fat (1440 calories) and 100 grams of carbohydrate (400 calories) for a total of 2040 calories. Nearly 71 percent of his calories were from fat—a percentage considerably higher than the typical American diet today, in which 40 to 50 percent of calories are from fat. It is not surprising then that the autopsy of Mr. Thompson at the age of 27 showed that he had marked atherosclerosis and coronary artery disease.

Since those days, many studies have shown that diets high in complex carbohydrates (starch and fiber) are linked with better control of blood glucose levels. As an added benefit, such diets can reduce serum cholesterol and triglyceride levels as well.

Today nutritional recommendations support a high-carbohydrate diet with proportions of fat and carbohydrate almost exactly the opposite of those prescribed for Mr. Thompson 60 years ago. The table below shows how the recommendations have changed over the years.

Percentage of calories from carbohydrate, protein and fat

Year	Carbohydrate	Protein	Fat
Before 1921	Starvation diets		
1921	20%	10%	70%
1950	40%	20%	40%
1979	50-60%	12-20%	30-35%
1986	55-60%	12-20%	25-30%

From 1921 to the 1950s the diet continued to be high in fat and low in carbohydrate, but there was little agreement on how best to implement these recommendations. In 1948, Dr. Frank Allen, a prominent diabetologist, speaking at the annual American Dietetic Association meeting, stated that most of the two million diabetics in the United States received little or no dietary treatment. He attributed this to the complicated methods used to calculate food intake and diets. Also, information about which foods to include and which to restrict was inconsistent, instructions given to patients were confusing, and diets were rarely adjusted to the individual's social, economic, or psychological circumstances. Because of these inconsistencies and confusion, a joint committee was appointed by the American Diabetes Association and the American Dietetic Association, and "exchange lists" were born.

When the exchange lists were first developed in 1951, the goal was to prepare a set of representative values for different food groups and to simplify meal planning.

One of the interesting aspects is the radical changes in recommendations for the use of vegetables. In light of today's knowledge, this seems strange, considering vegetables contain the least amount of carbohydrate and therefore have the smallest effect on blood glucose levels of any of the food groups.

Before 1921, "thrice-cooked" vegetables were recommended. This was to take advantage of their low carbohydrate content and to reduce it even further. Vegetables were cooked and drained three times to lower the carbohydrate content. After 1921, some nutritionists classified vegetables into lists containing approximately 3, 5, 9, and 12 percent carbohydrate, while others grouped them into lists of 5, 10, or 15 percent carbohydrate. With little uniformity, this percentage system was confusing to persons and hard to put into practical use.

The exchange lists of 1951 attempted to simplify this problem by grouping vegetables in "A" and "B" categories and by placing the vegetables that were high in carbohydrate into the list of bread exchanges. In 1951 it was reported "none of the other lists represents as major a change as this new classification of vegetables."

In 1971, the American Diabetes Association reviewed nutritional recommendations for people with diabetes and found it no longer necessary nor appropriate to continue the restriction of carbohydrate. Also, with fat in the diet beginning to be linked to the development of heart disease, they recommended reducing the percentage of calories from fat. This was a difficult idea for many people to understand and accept; it was practically the opposite of what they had been taught for years.

In 1976, the exchange lists were revised for the first time in 25 years. The major goal of that revision was to emphasize the need to reduce fat in the diet and to determine more accurately the total caloric intake. The meat list was divided into three groups—lean, medium, and high fat—making it easy to see at a glance which meats were the best choices. The milk list was based on skim or non-fat milk, and skim milk was recommended for use. The vegetable list was simplified, and all relatively low carbohydrate vegetables were grouped into one vegetable list, while the starchy vegetables remained on the bread list.

In 1986, a Task Force of the American Diabetes Association again updated the nutritional recommendations for individuals with diabetes. Based on these recommendations, the exchange lists were also revised to reflect nutrition as we understand it today. The emphasis is on a diet low in fat and higher in carbohydrate and fiber. In the new exchange lists, fiber values are given and a symbol indicates foods high in fiber. The exchange lists of 1986 also alert us to foods high in sodium.

Today, the diet for individuals with diabetes is less rigid and more flexible than it has been in the past. This is not because of less emphasis on meal planning; better methods of managing diabetes have reinforced the importance of attention to food intake if blood glucose levels are to be kept in the normal range.

However, today we are learning how to control glucose levels better, and this gives us more flexibility in meal planning. The goal continues to be the same: maintaining normal blood glucose and optimal fat levels. We hope this book will help you meet this goal.

Chapter Two
NUTRITION FOR THE FUTURE

L ifestyle has a strong influence on our health—and eating is an important part of lifestyle. Fortunately, most of us can choose what we eat. Awareness of the health benefits and risks associated with various foods leads to an important question: "How should we eat to stay healthy?"

It is becoming increasingly clear that the nutritional recommendations for persons with diabetes are part of a healthy lifestyle. In fact, everyone could benefit from making similar changes, and all of us could be the healthier for it.

Research has shown that control of certain dietary substances can reduce our risk of heart disease, high blood pressure, stroke, obesity, non-insulin-dependent diabetes, dental cavities, cirrhosis of the liver, and some forms of cancer (breast, colon, prostate, stomach, and esophagus). The nutritional recommendations made by the American Heart Association, American Cancer Society, and National Institutes of Cancer and stated in the Dietary Guidelines for Americans are very similar to the recommendations of the American Diabetes Association.

If your family's eating habits need to change because someone has developed diabetes, consider yourself lucky—not deprived. You now have a special reason to pay attention to planning meals and snacks that will help your family live better today and in the future. Eating wholesome, nutritionally healthy foods will be to everyone's advantage. What is of benefit for the individual with diabetes is of benefit to everyone in the family.

The new exchange lists reflect the latest scientific knowledge on nutrition and diabetes management and emphasize healthy eating for all Americans. A key feature is the positive approach to meal planning. The exchange lists now make it easier for individuals with diabetes to make healthy food choices.

What are the guidelines for good nutrition in diabetes? Here's an overview of some important nutrition recommendations and principles for persons who have diabetes.

Calories

It is important for all individuals to have a meal plan that meets their caloric requirements. Children and adolescents often require large numbers of calories in order to provide for their energy and growth requirement. They do NOT need a diet restricted in calories. Lean or normal weight adults also need a meal plan that provides enough calories for them to maintain their weight.

However, for some individuals, especially those with non-insulin-dependent diabetes, a meal plan that helps them lose weight may be important. It should not be so restricted in calories that you can't stick to it. Often even minor weight loss can help lower blood glucose levels and reduce the need for insulin or oral medication. Cutting back 500 calories from your daily intake will normally produce a gradual weight loss.

Carbohydrate

The amount of carbohydrate in your diet should ideally be 55 to 60 percent of your total calories. However, this should be individualized for your lifestyle. A high-fiber, low-fat diet is recommended. Substituting foods that contain fiber for foods that are more refined may also be helpful. See chapters 13 and 35 for ideas on how to do this.

Some individuals may also be able to use modest amounts of sucrose and other refined sugars in their meal plans without it affecting their blood glucose control. Different carbohydrates affect blood glucose levels differently, but it is not a matter of sugar versus starches. However, if you choose to eat foods containing sugar you must realize the portion sizes will probably be small. Most foods containing sugar will have a considerable amount of calories packed into a relatively small serving size!

Second, you need to know how to use sugar foods in your meal plan correctly. Generally foods containing sugar (ice cream, cookies, cakes, etc.) are substituted for starch/bread or fruit exchanges. See chapter 12 for some ideas on how to do this. There are few foods you can eat "all you want" or in very large portions without affecting your blood glucose control.

The best advice that can be given anyone (with or without diabetes) is the more foods containing sugar that can be avoided, the better. Sugar calories are called "empty calories," meaning that they provide no important nutrients, such as vitamins, minerals, or fiber. They just add calories.

Protein

At present we can't say what the ideal percentages of calories from protein should be for a healthy meal plan. Researchers are beginning to wonder if diets too high in protein contribute to the development of kidney disease, and some are beginning to caution individuals to eat less protein. The majority of Americans consume two to three times as much protein as they actually need. This is also true for individuals with diabetes as well.

Fat

People with diabetes seem to have a particularly high risk for developing heart and blood vessel disease. The three main risk factors for this are high blood cholesterol levels, high blood pressure, and smoking. Diets high in fat, especially saturated fat, and cholesterol contribute to an elevated blood cholesterol. By cutting back on fat and cholesterol you can usually lower your blood fat levels. The recommendation is that 30 percent or less of your calories come from fat and that cholesterol be limited to 300 mg/dl day. Try to replace saturated fats with unsaturated fats. See chapter 9 for ideas on how to do this. However, it is again important that this recommendation be individualized for you.

There is also some evidence that unsaturated fats from fish, called "omega-35," may be beneficial in lowering triglycerides and cholesterol. Fish found in cold waters, "fatty" fish, and shellfish are good sources of these fish oils and should be eaten a couple of times a week.

Salt (Sodium)

Too much sodium is a prime suspect in high blood pressure, especially in persons who are genetically susceptible to high blood pressure. Also, high blood pressure seems to be related to earlier onset of diabetic complications. Therefore, it seems wise to restrict sodium in the diet to 1,000 mg per 1,000 calories or no more than 3,000 mg of sodium per day (about the equivalent of a teaspoon of salt).

Non-nutritive Sweeteners

Non-nutritive sweeteners made from aspartame and saccharine are believed to be safe. It is recommended that they be used in moderation and that a variety of sweeteners be used to lessen the chance of consuming too much of any one product. See chapter 33 for more information.

Alcohol

Everyone should be aware of the dangers of too much alcohol, but people with diabetes should also be aware that alcohol can cause hypoglycemia (low blood sugar), especially if consumed without food. Alcohol can also be high in calories. Nonetheless, if you choose to drink an occasional alcoholic beverage, you can usually do so safely. See chapter xx for guidelines.

Vitamins and Minerals

People who have diabetes do not have any special needs for vitamins and minerals that are different from anyone else.

Goals of Meal Planning

Meal planning is intended to help you keep your blood glucose under as good control as is possible and to keep blood fats (cholesterol and triglycerides) in an ideal range.

For people using insulin, the best way to do this is to eat as consistently as possible—approximately the same amount of food at the same times each day. By eating consistently and by monitoring your blood glucose to see what is happening, insulin therapy can usually be integrated into your food habits.

For people being controlled by diet alone the best way to help you meet your goals is by weight management.

As you think about healthy eating and how your family will follow the nutritional guidelines for individuals with diabetes, keep these goals in mind:

good food, good health, and good taste.

Too often we equate a diet rich in fat, cholesterol, sugar, calories, and salt with good tasting food. However, this is not necessarily true. Healthy food does taste good!

Poor eating habits are risk factors for many of the chronic diseases affecting Americans today. The happy truth is that with gradual and moderate changes in our eating habits, we can live much better and probably longer—and we'll look better, too.

Chapter Three
EXCHANGE LISTS
MAKE MEAL PLANNING
EASIER AND ADD VARIETY

The exchange system has been developed to make meal planning for individuals with diabetes easier. The revised exchange lists reflect the latest scientific knowledge on nutrition and diabetes management and emphasize the value of healthy eating for all Americans.

Exchange lists are based on the amount of carbohydrate, protein, and fat in foods. These nutrients provide calories and require insulin to be metabolized. Each exchange has approximately the same number of calories and carbohydrate, protein, and fat content as other foods on the same list. Therefore, a food, in the amount listed, can be exchanged for any other food on the same list.

An "exchange" is a measured amount of food selected from a group of foods that are similar to it. **Exchange Lists for Meal Planning** groups foods into six lists (exchange lists), and the foods within a group have approximately the same nutritive value. Many foods fall into one of six groups:

Starch/breads
Meat and meat substitutes
Vegetables
Fruits
Milk
Fat

The use of exchange lists allows you to select a variety of foods without calculating the value of each one.

In addition to the six lists of basic foods there are several other categories:

- Free-foods—any food or drink with less than 20 calories per serving;
- "Combination" foods such as casseroles, soups, and pizza;
- "Special occasion" foods, including ice cream, cake, cookies, simple desserts.

Persons with diabetes now have more food variety to spice up their lives. The "mix and match" or "trade off" feature within the same food group will make it easier to select foods from a wider variety of foods. The added lists will also make it easier to add variety to meal planning.

A meal plan tells you how many servings from each list you can select for each meal and for snacks. It is important that you have a meal plan individualized for your caloric and lifestyle needs. Your meal plan is your guide as to what—and when—you should be eating throughout the day.

Exchange lists for many common foods are included in *Exchange Lists for Meal Planning,* published by the American Dietetic Association. They are not repeated here. The following expanded exchange lists apply the same principles to a greater variety of foods, making it easier to add variety to your meal plan.

Chapter Four
STARCH/BREAD EXCHANGES

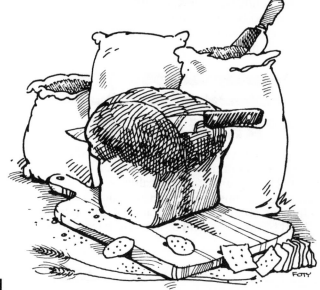

Individuals with diabetes are encouraged to increase the percentage of calories in their meal plan that come from carbohydrates, while reducing calories from fat. The recommendation is to increase carbohydrates, especially those that also contain fiber. Many foods that contain carbohydrates and fiber are found on the starch/bread list. You will notice this is now the first list. This was done to draw attention to the importance of these foods in your meal plan.

If you are unsure of the correct portion size for bread products, a one-ounce portion by weight is a good rule of thumb. For example, a one-ounce hamburger or frankfurter bun or a one-ounce slice of French bread is one starch/bread exchange and a two-ounce bun is two starch/bread exchanges. One-half cup of cereal, grain or pasta is another ground rule for starch foods when you are unsure of the portion size.

Soups can most easily be counted as starch/bread exchanges. A cup of broth-type soup, such as chicken noodle or vegetable beef, is one starch/bread exchange. A bowl of soup usually is closer to 2 cups and would be counted as 2 starch/breads. One cup of a cream soup is one starch/bread exchange plus one fat exchange.

Starch/bread and meat exchanges also can be used to count

casseroles and hotdishes. If you are unsure of the make-up of a combination dish, count one cup as two starch/bread exchanges plus two medium fat meat exchanges. Depending on the ingredients, the casserole may also include a fat or a vegetable exchange. For example, one cup of chili, beef stew, or macaroni and beef casserole is two starch/bread and two medium fat meat exchanges. One cup of tuna noodle casserole containing cream soup is one fat, two starch/bread and two medium fat meat exchanges.

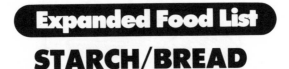

Expanded Food List
STARCH/BREAD

Food value: The following foods contain approximately 15 grams of carbohydrate, 3 grams of protein, a trace of fat (approximately 1/2 to 1 gram), and 80 calories. Whole grain breads and crackers average 2 grams of fiber per serving. Cereals containing fiber and starchy vegetables average 3 grams of fiber per serving. Bran cereals, dried beans, peas, and lentils will have 4 to 8 grams of fiber per serving.

Food	Quantity	Exchanges
Cereals/Grains/Pasta		
Cereals:		
Bran Chex	1/2 cup	1 starch/bread
Raisin Bran	1/2 cup	1 starch/bread
100% Bran	1/3 cup	1 starch/bread
40% Bran	1/2 cup	1 starch/bread
Cheerios	1 cup	1 starch/bread
Honey Nut Cheerios	3/4 cup	1 starch/bread
Corn Bran	1/2 cup	1 starch/bread
Corn Chex	2/3 cup	1 starch/bread
Corn Flakes	3/4 cup	1 starch/bread
Cream of Rice	3/4 cup	1 starch/bread
Crispy Wheat 'n Raisins	1/2 cup	1 starch/bread
Farina	1/2 cup	1 starch/bread
Fiber One	1/2 cup	1 starch/bread
Granola	1/4 cup	1 starch/bread 1 fat
Malt-O-Meal	1/2 cup	1 starch/bread
Maypo, cooked	1/3 cup	1 starch/bread
Nutri-Grain	1/2 cup	1 starch/bread

Food	Quantity	Exchanges
Oatflakes	1/2 cup	1 starch/bread
Oatmeal	1/2 cup	1 starch/bread
Puffed Corn	1 cup	1 starch/bread
Puffed Rice	1¼ cup	1 starch/bread
Puffed Wheat	1½ cup	1 starch/bread
Rice Chex	3/4 cup	1 starch/bread
Roman Meal	1/3 cup	1 starch/bread
Shredded Wheat	1 large biscuit	1 starch/bread
Shredded Wheat, spoon size	16 pieces (3/4 oz.)	1 starch/bread
Special K	1 cup	1 starch/bread
Total	1/2 cup	1 starch/bread
Wheat Bran, unprocessed, unsweetened	1/2 cup	1 starch/bread
Wheat Chex	1/2 cup	1 starch/bread
Wheat Germ	3 Tbsp.	1 starch/bread
Wheaties	3/4 cup	1 starch/bread
Barley	1/3 cup	1 starch/bread
Buckwheat groats (Kasha), cooked	1/3 cup	1 starch/bread
Couscous	1/3 cup	1 starch/bread
Cornstarch	2 Tbsp	1 starch/bread
Farfel	3 Tbsp.	1 starch/bread
Flour	3 Tbsp.	1 starch/bread
Hominy, cooked	1/2 cup	1 starch/bread
Miller's bran	1/4 cup	1/2 starch/bread
Rice, brown, cooked	1/3 cup	1 starch/bread
Rice, fried	1/2 cup	1 starch/bread 2 fat
Rice, instant, cooked	1/3 cup	1 starch/bread
Rice, long grain and wild	1/3 cup	1 starch/bread
Scrapple	1 oz.	1 starch/bread 1 fat
Somen or udon (noodles), cooked	1/2 cup	1 starch/bread
Tapioca, dry	2 Tbsp.	1 starch/bread
Starchy Vegetables:		
Chestnuts, roasted	4 large, 6 small	1 starch/bread

Food	Quantity	Exchanges
Corn, cream style	1/3 cup	1 starch/bread
Corn pudding	1/2 cup	1 starch/bread 1 fat
Malanga, boiled	1/2 cup	1 starch/bread
Onion rings, frozen	4 average	1 starch/bread 2 fat
Blackeyed peas, canned	1/2 cup	1 starch/bread
Cowpeas, frozen, boiled	1/3 cup	1 starch/bread
Parsnips, cooked	1/2 cup, sliced	1 starch/bread
Potatoes:		
Au gratin	1/2 cup	1 starch/bread 1 fat
Dinner fries, cottage fries	2 oz.	1 starch/bread 1 fat
Flakes, as prepared	1/2 cup	1 starch/bread 1 fat
French fried, frozen, heated in oven	3/4 cup	1 starch/bread 1 fat
French fried, restaurant	1/2 cup	1 starch/bread 1 fat
Hashed brown, home prepared	1/2 cup	1 starch/bread 2 fat
Frozen potato puffs, pan-fried	1/2 cup	1 starch/bread 1 fat
Scalloped	1/2 cup	1 starch/bread 1 fat
Stix or shoestrings	3/4 cup (1 oz.)	1 starch/bread 2 fat
Tater-tots	1/2 cup	1 starch/bread 1 fat
Rutabaga, boiled	3/4 cup	1 starch/bread
Salsify or oyster plant, cubed, cooked	3/4 cup	1 starch/bread
Green soybeans, boiled	1/2 cup	1/2 starch/bread 1 med. fat meat
Succotash	1/2 cup	1 starch/bread
Sweet potato, baked	1/2 average, 5″ long, 2″ diameter	1 starch/bread
Taro root, diced, raw	1/2 cup	1 starch/bread
Mixed vegetables	3/4 cup	1 starch/bread
Water chestnuts,	1/2 cup	1 starch/bread

Food	Quantity	Exchanges
Breads:		
Banana bread	1 slice (1/16 of a loaf)	1 starch/bread 1 fat
Blueberry muffin	1 average	1 starch/bread 1 fat
Boston brown bread	1 slice 3" round × 1/2"	1 starch/bread
Brown and Serve rolls	1 average	1 starch/bread
Bread crumbs, dry	3 Tbsp.	1 starch/bread
Bread, home baked or unsliced	1 oz.	1 starch/bread
Bread sticks, 8" long, 1/2" diameter	2 sticks	1 starch/bread
Bread sticks, 4" long, 1/4" diameter	6 sticks	1 starch/bread
Cocktail or party rye bread	3 slices	1 starch/bread
Corn pone	1 cake (1½ oz.)	1 starch/bread 1/2 fat
Croissants	1 (1½ oz.)	1½ starch/bread 2 fat
Crumpet	1	1 starch/bread
French bread	3" slice	1 starch/bread
French toast	1 slice	1 starch/bread 1/2 med. fat meat
Kaiser or hard roll *p.103 sugar ½*	1	1 starch/bread
Muffin	1 average	1 starch/bread 1 fat
Pan/dinner roll	1 average	1 starch/bread
Patty shell	1	1 starch/bread 3 fat
Pocket bread, 4½" diameter	1	1 starch/bread
Pocket bread, 6" diameter	1	1 starch/bread
Popover	1 small	1 starch/bread 1 fat
Rice cakes, crispy	2 cakes	1 starch/bread 2 fat
Spoon bread	3½ oz.	1 starch/bread 2 fat

Food	Quantity	Exchanges
Tea breads (pumpkin, cranberry, etc.)	1 slice (1½ oz.)	1½ starch/bread 1 fat
Tostada shell	2 average	1 starch/bread 1 fat
Crackers:		
Animal	8	1 starch/bread
Cheese Nips	20	1 starch/bread 1 fat
Cheez-Its	27	1 starch/bread 1 fat
Goldfish	1/3 cup 1 handful	1 starch/bread 1 fat
Matzo, 6" diameter	1 (3/4 oz.)	1 starch/bread
Matzo crackers, thin, 1½" square	7	1 starch/bread
Melba toast, oblong	5	1 starch/bread
Melba toast, round	10	1 starch/bread
Ritz, Hi Ho, etc.	6	1 starch/bread 1 fat
Rusks	2	1 starch/bread
Rye wafers	3	1 starch/bread
Ry Krisp	3 triple crackers	1 starch/bread
Sesame snack	8	1 starch/bread 1 fat
Skittle chips	10 (1 oz.)	1 starch/bread 1½ fat
Sociables	11 (1 oz.)	1 starch/bread 1 fat
Triscuit wafers	5 (3/4 oz.)	1 starch/bread 1 fat
Uneeda biscuit	4 biscuits (3/4 oz.)	1 starch/bread
Waverly wafers	5 wafers (3/4 oz.)	1 starch/bread
Wheat thins	12 (1 oz.)	1 starch/bread
Wheatbury Wheat Snacks	15 crackers	1 starch/bread
Zwiebach	3 (3/4 oz.)	1 starch/bread
Pancakes, frozen, microwave	1	1 starch/bread

Food	Quantity	Exchanges
Snack foods:		
Bugles	30 (1 oz.)	1 starch/bread 2 fat
Cheese puffed balls	1 oz.	1 starch/bread 2 fat
Cheese twists	1 oz.	1 starch/bread 2 fat
Cheetos	3/4 oz.	1 starch/bread 1 fat
Cornnuts	3/4 oz.	1 starch/bread 1 fat
Corn chips, Fritos, Doritos	3/4 oz.	1 starch/bread 1 fat
Chicken egg roll	1/2 average	1 starch/bread 1 fat
Doo Dads	3/4 oz.	1 starch/bread 1 fat
Potato chips	3/4 oz.	1 starch/bread 1 fat
Popcorn, microwave	3 cups popped	1 starch/bread 2 fat
Pretzels	3/4 oz.	1 starch/bread
Very thin twisted	4	1 starch/bread
Pretzelettes	12	1 starch/bread
Very thin sticks	67	1 starch/bread
Won ton, fried	3	1 starch/bread 4 fat
Soups:		
Cream of asparagus, prepared with milk	1 cup	1 starch/bread 1/2 skim milk 1 fat
Baked bean with bacon, prepared with water	1 cup	1½ starch/bread 1 fat
Bean with frankfurters, prepared with water	1 cup	1½ starch/bread 1 fat
Beef chili, prepared with water	1 cup	1½ starch/bread 1 fat
Tomato beef with noodles, prepared with water	1 cup	1½ starch/bread 1 fat
Beef noodle, prepared with water	1 cup	1 starch/bread

Food	Quantity	Exchanges
Chicken noodle, prepared with water	1 cup	1 starch/bread
Chicken vegetable, prepared with water	1 cup	1 starch/bread
Chicken with rice, prepared with water	1 cup	1 starch/bread
Minestrone, prepared with water	1 cup	1 starch/bread
Onion, prepared with water	1 cup	1 starch/bread
Tomato with rice, prepared with water	1 cup	1 starch/bread
Turkey noodle, prepared with water	1 cup	1 starch/bread
Vegetable with beef, prepared with water	1 cup	1 starch/bread
Vegetarian vegetable, prepared with water	1 cup	1 starch/bread
Cream of celery, prepared with milk	1 cup	1 starch/bread 2 fat
Cream of chicken, prepared with milk	1 cup	1 starch/bread 2 fat
Cheese, prepared with milk	1 cup	1 starch/bread 3 fat
Chunky soups, ready ready to serve	1 10¾ oz. can	1 starch/bread 1 vegetable 1 med. fat meat
Cream of mushroom, prepared with milk	1 cup	1 starch/bread 3 fat
Clam chowder, prepared with milk	1 cup	1 starch/bread 1 fat
Oyster stew, prepared with milk	1 cup	1 starch/bread 1 fat
Cream of potato, prepared with milk	1 cup	1 starch/bread 1 fat
Tomato, prepared with milk	1 cup	1 starch/bread 1 fat
Split pea with ham, prepared with water	1 cup	2 starch/bread 1 fat
Won ton soup, homemade	1 cup	1 starch/bread 2½ med. fat meat
Waffles, Eggo	1 waffle	1 starch/bread 1 fat

Word List

Bulgur: Whole wheat berry that is parboiled, dried and broken up. Cooks very quickly.

Cassava: Also known as the yucca root. It has a large, starchy root. The starch derived from the root of this plant is used to make tapioca. Bitter odor that disappears upon cooking.

Chestnuts: A nut that has a hard, brown outer shell and an inner shell that protects the kernel. To shell make a deep x on the flat side. Cover with boiling water and simmer 2 to 3 minutes. Drain 2 to 3 nuts at a time; pull off shells and inner skins. To roast make a deep x on flat side; roast in a 450° oven for 15-20 minutes. To roast in a fireplace, place nuts on edge of open fire or in a long handle popcorn basket. Shake over fire until they pop.

Couscous: Precooked hard-cracked granules of semolina wheat. It can be cooked quickly by a soak and steam method.

Malanga: Large herbs grown in the tropics for edible root.

Salsify: Also known as oyster plant. It has a parsnip appearance an oyster flavor.

Succotash: A dish of North American Indian origin. It consists of corn and beans.

Taro root: Commonly used in Hawaii and eaten in the form of poi. Cooked taro ranges in color from purple to cream.

Chapter Five
MEAT AND MEAT SUBSTITUTES

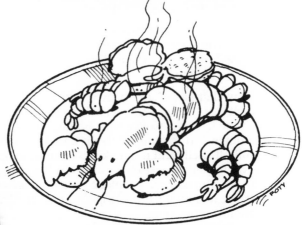

Meat portion sizes are based on cooked meat with the fat and bone removed. Because meat portions are difficult to estimate, it is helpful to weigh meat. This is especially important when using meats you have not used before.

For persons with diabetes, it is important to reduce the total fat content of the diet. This can be done by using lean meat choices or using food preparation methods that eliminate fat in the cooking process and by watching your portion sizes.

There are three meat lists: lean meat, medium-fat meat, and high-fat meat. The foods listed contain approximately the same amount of protein but are divided into the three lists based on their fat content.

Expanded Food List
LEAN MEAT

Food value: The following foods contain approximately 7 grams of protein, 3 grams of fat and 55 calories. Each is equal to one lean meat exchange.

Food	Quantity	Exchanges
Beef		
Beef jerky	1/2 oz.	1 lean meat
Cubed flank steak	1 oz.	1 lean meat

Food	Quantity	Exchanges
Dried chipped beef	1 oz.	1 lean meat
Family steak	1 oz.	1 lean meat
Filet mignon	1 oz.	1 lean meat
Kabob cubes	1 oz.	1 lean meat
Loin steak, boneless	1 oz.	1 lean meat
London broil	1 oz.	1 lean meat
Round roast or steak	1 oz.	1 lean meat
Sandwich steaks	1 oz.	1 lean meat
Shank	1 oz.	1 lean meat
Skirt steak	1 oz.	1 lean meat
Stew meat	1 oz.	1 lean meat
Sweetbreads	1 oz.	1 lean meat
Tenderloin tips	1 oz.	1 lean meat
Very lean ground round or sirloin (90% lean)	1 oz.	1 lean meat

Cheese—Low fat, containing 3 grams or less of fat per ounce. (See section on Cheese Guidelines.)

Low fat cottage cheese (2%)	1 oz.	1 lean meat
Regular cottage cheese (4%)	1 oz.	1 lean meat
Chef's Delight	1 oz.	1 lean meat
Diet cheeses:	1 oz.	1 lean meat
Calorie Wise (Kraft) cheese spread	1 oz.	1 lean meat
Countdown (Fisher)	1 oz.	1 lean meat
Light 'n Lively American Pasteurized process cheese (Kraft)	1 oz.	1 lean meat
Lite-Line (Bordon)	1 oz.	1 lean meat
Weight Watchers low fat cheese slices	1 oz.	1 lean meat
Farmer's	1 oz.	1 lean meat
Gammelost (Norwegian strong)	1 oz.	1 lean meat
Hoop cheese	1 oz.	1 lean meat
Laughing Cow skim milk cheese wedges	1 (3/4 oz.)	1 lean meat
May Bud skim milk (Purity)	1 oz.	1 lean meat
Pot cheese	1/4 cup	1 lean meat
Ricotta, made with part skim milk	2 Tbsp.	1 lean meat

Food	Quantity	Exchanges
Sap Sago	1 oz.	1 lean meat
St. Otho	1 oz.	1 lean meat
Tasty Brand Imitation Process Cheese Loaf or cheese spread	1 oz.	1 lean meat
Tilsit, slim	1 oz.	1 lean meat
Weight Watchers Lo-fat cheese slices	1 oz.	1 lean meat
Wisconsin Skim Milk Cheese (Purity)	1 oz.	1 lean meat

Egg

Food	Quantity	Exchanges
Egg whites	2	1 lean meat
Egg substitute	1/4 cup	1 lean meat

Fish

Food	Quantity	Exchanges
Clams	1/2 cup	1 lean meat
Clams, hard shell	3/4 large	1 lean meat
Clams, soft shell	2 large	1 lean meat
Crab, lobster	1/3 cup (1 oz.)	1 lean meat
Crab meat, canned	1/4 cup	1 lean meat
Crayfish	2 oz.	1 lean meat
Frog legs	3 medium (1 oz.)	1 lean meat
Mussels	2 oz.	1 lean meat
Octopus	1 oz.	1 lean meat
Oysters, raw meat only	5 average	1 lean meat
Squid	1 oz.	1 lean meat
Tuna	1/4 cup	1 lean meat

Game

Food	Quantity	Exchanges
Rabbit	1 oz.	1 lean meat
Squirrel	1 oz.	1 lean meat
Venison	1 oz.	1 lean meat

Lamb

Food	Quantity	Exchanges
Cubes	1 oz.	1 lean meat
Shish Kabob	1 oz.	1 lean meat
Shoulder roast	1 oz.	1 lean meat
Sirloin roast	1 oz.	1 lean meat

Pork

Food	Quantity	Exchanges
Leg (fresh ham)	1 oz.	1 lean meat
Canned ham	1 oz.	1 lean meat

Food	Quantity	Exchanges
Cured ham	1 oz.	1 lean meat
Poultry		
Capon	1 oz.	1 lean meat
Chicken, diced	1/4 cup	1 lean meat
Chicken livers, simmered	4 average	1 lean meat
Chicken, canned	1 oz.	1 lean meat
Smoked turkey breast	1 oz.	1 lean meat
Turkey ham	1 oz.	1 lean meat
Veal		
Chop	1 oz.	1 lean meat
Roast	1 oz.	1 lean meat
Steak cutlet	1 oz.	1 lean meat

Expanded Food List
MEDIUM-FAT MEAT

Food value: The following foods contain approximately 7 grams of protein, 5 grams of fat and 75 calories. Each is one medium-fat meat exchange unless otherwise specified. Most beef and pork roasts or steaks fall into this category.

Food	Quantity	Exchanges
Beef		
Blade steak or pot roast	1 oz.	1 med. fat meat
Boneless chuck steak or roast, well trimmed	1 oz.	1 med. fat meat
Club steak	1 oz.	1 med. fat meat
Meat balls	1 oz.	1 med. fat meat
New York strip steak	1 oz.	1 med. fat meat
Porterhouse steak	1 oz.	1 med. fat meat
Rib roast	1 oz.	1 med. fat meat
Shoulder steak	1 oz.	1 med. fat meat
Sirloin tip roast	1 oz.	1 med. fat meat
T-bone steak	1 oz.	1 med. fat meat
Ground beef, drained	1/2 cup cooked	3 med. fat meat

Cheeses with 3 to 5 grams of fat per ounce should be used in place of a medium-fat meat. The saturated fat and cholesterol content of those cheeses are similar to 1 ounce of medium-fat meat.

Food	Quantity	Exchanges
American Cheese spread	1 oz.	1 med. fat meat
Cheez Kisses	1 oz.	1 med. fat meat
Cheez Whiz cheese spread	1 oz.	1 med. fat meat
Cheriss (similar to Baby Swiss)	1 oz.	1 med. fat meat
Feta	1 oz.	1 med. fat meat
Green River skim milk cheese (Lucerne)	1 oz.	1 med. fat meat
Mozzarella, part skim	1 oz.	1 med. fat meat
Mozzarella, pizza (Kraft)	1 oz.	1 med. fat meat
Neufchâtel	1 oz. (3 Tbsp.)	1 med. fat meat
Olympia diet cheese	1 oz.	1 med. fat meat
Parmesan cheese	1 oz.	1 med. fat meat
Philadelphia Light (Kraft) cream cheese	1 oz.	1 med. fat meat
Ricotta, whole milk	1 oz.	1 med. fat meat
Skim American (Borden)	1 oz.	1 med. fat meat
Slimline (Borden)	1 oz.	1 med. fat meat
Slimost Lowfat Colby	1 oz.	1 med. fat meat
String cheese	1 oz.	1 med. fat meat
Tivoli Danalette (a low fat Danbo cheese)	1 oz.	1 med. fat meat
Velveeta loaf and spread	1 oz.	1 med. fat meat
Weight Watchers natural part skim milk cheese	1 oz.	1 med. fat meat

Eggs

Food	Quantity	Exchanges
Egg omelet	2 eggs	2 med. fat meat 1 fat
Cheese souffle	4 oz.	1 med. fat meat 1/2 milk 3 fat

Fish

Food	Quantity	Exchanges
Anchovy fillets, drained	9	1 med. fat meat
Caviar, fish roe	1 oz.	1 med. fat meat
Deviled crab	2 oz.	1/2 starch/bread 1 med. fat meat
Pickled herring	1 oz.	1 med. fat meat
Mackerel	1 oz.	1 med. fat meat
Oysters, fried, breaded	3 oz.	1 med. fat meat 1 starch/bread 1 fat

Food	Quantity	Exchanges
Rainbow trout	1 oz.	1 med. fat meat
Sablefish	1 oz.	1 med. fat meat
Salmon, Chinook	1 oz.	1 med. fat meat
Shrimp, French fried, breaded	4 oz.	1 starch/bread 3 med. fat meat
Smelt	1 oz.	1 med. fat meat
Sticks	4	1½ starch/bread 1 med. fat meat
Lamb		
Chops, rib or shoulder	1 oz.	1 med. fat meat
Crown roast	1 oz.	1 med. fat meat
Leg, roast and chops	1 oz.	1 med. fat meat
Steaks	1 oz.	1 med. fat meat
Pork		
Butterfly pork chops	1 oz.	1 med. fat meat
Crown roast of pork	1 oz.	1 med. fat meat
Cubes	1 oz.	1 med. fat meat
Cutlets	1 oz.	1 med. fat meat
Loin roast	1 oz.	1 med. fat meat
Sirloin chops	1 oz.	1 med. fat meat
Smoked pork chops	1 oz.	1 med. fat meat
Tenderloin	1 oz.	1 med. fat meat
Beans		
Tofu, soybean curd	3 oz. (1 piece, 2½″ x 2¾″ × 1″)	1 med. fat meat

Expanded Food List
HIGH-FAT MEAT

Food value: The following foods contain approximately 7 grams of protein, 8 grams of fat and 100 calories. Each is equal to one high-fat meat exchange unless otherwise specified. Prime grades of meat, meat with high fat content, most cheeses, cold cuts, frankfurters and sausages are in this category.

Food	Quantity	Exchanges
Beef		
Prime rib roasts and steaks	1 oz.	1 high fat meat

Food	Quantity	Exchanges

Cheeses with 6 to 8 grams of fat per ounce are made from whole milk. They contain a large amount of saturated fat and cholesterol. (See section on Cheese Guidelines.)

Black Diamond	1 oz.	1 high fat meat
Blue	1 oz.	1 high fat meat
Brick	1 oz.	1 high fat meat
Brie	1 oz.	1 high fat meat
Camembert	1 oz.	1 high fat meat
Caraway	1 oz.	1 high fat meat
Barbecue ribs	1 oz.	1 high fat meat
Blade cut chuck roast	1 oz.	1 high fat meat
Brisket	1 oz.	1 high fat meat
Hamburger, more than 20% fat	1 oz.	1 high fat meat
Ribs	1 oz.	1 high fat meat
Short ribs	1 oz.	1 high fat meat
Lean 'n Tasty (Beef breakfast strips)	2 strips	1 high fat meat

Cheeses with 6 to 8 grams of low cholesterol fat per pound (filled skim milk cheese) are similar in total fat to regular cheese but low in cholesterol and saturated fat. (See section on Cheese Guidelines.)

Cheezola (Fisher), corn oil, cholesterol free	1 oz.	1 high fat meat
Dorman's Low-chol or Tilsiter cheese	1 oz.	1 high fat meat
Hickory Farms, Longhorn Lyte	1 oz.	1 high fat meat
Hickory Farms, Smokey Lyte	1 oz.	1 high fat meat
Lorraine Swiss	1 oz.	1 high fat meat
Merrywood Farm's Nu Trend cheeses:	1 oz.	1 high fat meat
Caraway Snack	1 oz.	1 high fat meat
Onion Snack	1 oz.	1 high fat meat
Hot 'N Spicy	1 oz.	1 high fat meat
Mild 'N Mellow	1 oz.	1 high fat meat
Hickory Smoked	1 oz.	1 high fat meat
Mini-Cholesterol	1 oz.	1 high fat meat
Scandic Cholesterol Free Cheese	1 oz.	1 high fat meat

Food	Quantity	Exchanges
Cheddar, Natural and Pasteurized Process	1 oz.	1 high fat meat
Cheshire	1 oz.	1 high fat meat
Colby	1 oz.	1 high fat meat
Curds	2 Tbsp.	1 high fat meat
Edam	1 oz.	1 high fat meat
Fontina	1 oz.	1 high fat meat
Gouda	1 oz.	1 high fat meat
Gruyere	1 oz.	1 high fat meat
Jarlsberg	1 oz.	1 high fat meat
Limburger	1 oz.	1 high fat meat
Longhorn	1 oz.	1 high fat meat
Monterey Jack	1 oz.	1 high fat meat
Mozzarella, whole milk	1 oz.	1 high fat meat
Muenster	1 oz.	1 high fat meat
Port du Salut	1 oz.	1 high fat meat
Provolone	1 oz.	1 high fat meat
Romano	1 oz.	1 high fat meat
Roquefort	1 oz.	1 high fat meat
Swiss, natural and process	1 oz.	1 high fat meat
Tilsit, regular	1 oz.	1 high fat meat
Pasteurized Process:		
American or American cheese food	1 oz.	1 high fat meat
Cold pack American cheese	1 oz.	1 high fat meat
Pimiento	1 oz.	1 high fat meat
Swiss or Swiss cheese food	1 oz.	1 high fat meat
Fish		
Eel	2 oz.	1 high fat meat 1 fat
Fried fish fillets	2 fillets (2 oz. total)	1 high fat meat 1½ bread
Shrimp sticks	5 sticks (2 oz. total)	1½ starch/bread 1 high fat meat
Luncheon Meats		
Blood sausage	1 oz.	1 high fat meat
Bologna	1 oz.	1 high fat meat
Bratwurst	1 oz.	1 high fat meat

Food	Quantity	Exchanges
Braunschweiger	1 oz.	1 high fat meat
Cocktail wiener	1 oz.	1 high fat meat
Deviled ham, canned	1 oz.	1 high fat meat
Head cheese	1 oz.	1 high fat meat
Knockwurst	1 oz.	1 high fat meat
Liverwurst	1 oz.	1 high fat meat
Pastrami	1 oz.	1 high fat meat
Pepperoni	1 oz.	1 high fat meat
Polish sausage	1 oz.	1 high fat meat
Salami	1 oz.	1 high fat meat
Spam	1 oz.	1 high fat meat
Thuringer	1 oz.	1 high fat meat
Treet	1 oz.	1 high fat meat
Pork		
Bacon	2 slices	1 high fat meat
Barbecue ribs	1 oz.	1 high fat meat
Cocktail wieners	3	1 high fat meat
Country ribs	1 oz.	1 high fat meat
Country style ham	1 oz.	1 high fat meat
Frankfurters	1 oz.	1 high fat meat
Fresh pork belly	1 oz.	1 high fat meat
Hock, smoked	1 oz.	1 high fat meat
Pig's feet	1 oz.	1 high fat meat
Sausage, bulk patties or link	1 oz.	1 high fat meat
Sizzlean breakfast strips	2 strips	1 high fat meat 1 fat
Spareribs	1 oz.	1 high fat meat
Vienna sausages	3 small	1 high fat meat

Nuts—A one-ounce serving of most nuts is counted as 1 high-fat meat plus 1 fat exchange or as 1 medium-fat meat plus 2 fat exchanges. A half-ounce serving could be counted as 1 high-fat meat exchange. Nuts in very small amounts are counted as fat exchanges. See the fat exchange list for portion sizes.

Food	Quantity	Exchanges
Cashews	14-15 (1 oz.)	1 med. fat meat 2 fat
Macadamia	12 med. (1 oz.)	1 med. fat meat 2 fat

Food	Quantity	Exchanges
Peanuts	1/4 cup (1 oz.)	1 med. fat meat 2 fat
Pine nuts (Pignolias)	1/4 cup (1 oz.)	1 med. fat meat 2 fat
Pistachio	60 nuts (1 oz.)	1 med. fat meat 2 fat
Walnuts	16-20 halves (1 oz.)	1 med. fat meat 2 fat
Mixed	16-24 (1 oz.)	1 med. fat meat 2 fat
Peanut butter	1 Tbsp.	1 high fat meat
Sunflower, pumpkin or **squash seeds**	1/4 cup	1 med. fat meat 1 fat

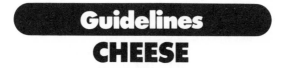

Guidelines

CHEESE

Cheese is a nutritious food; it provides protein, calcium, vitamin A, and other nutrients. However, cheese generally provides more fat than an equal portion of meat. The form of fat is predominantly saturated. In addition, cholesterol is found in cheese. How much fat and cholesterol a cheese contains depends on the type of milk used in its production. Milk used may be extra rich, whole, 2% or skim and may have butterfat (milkfat) added as well.

Cheese is also a relatively high sodium food, containing approximately 200 milligrams of sodium per ounce. Processed cheeses contain twice as much sodium (400 milligrams per ounce).

The fat content of cheese, if listed on the label, is indicated in one of two ways: grams of fat per ounce or by percent of fat. The percent of fat is equal to the grams of fat per 100 grams (3½ ounces) of cheese.

The following guidelines can help you select cheese. The recommendations are based on the grams of fat per ounce of cheese.

- Cheese with less than 1 gram of fat per ounce:

   Made with skim milk, these cheeses are included on the lean meat list.

- Cheese with 1 to 2 grams of fat per ounce:

   These cheeses, made primarily from skim milk, have a slightly higher fat content. They are still included on the lean meat list.

- Cheese with 3 to 5 grams of fat per ounce:

  The saturated fat and cholesterol content of these cheeses is similar to 1 ounce of medium fat meat.

- Cheese with 6 to 8 grams of fat per ounce:

  These cheeses are made from whole milk and contain a large amount of saturated fat and cholesterol. They are included on the high fat meat exchange list. Total fat is more than a teaspoon per ounce of cheese.

- Cheese with 6 to 8 grams of low cholesterol fat per ounce (filled skim milk cheese):

  Though similar in total fat to regular cheese, filled cheese is low in cholesterol and saturated fat. However, it is still included on the high fat meat list because of the total fat content. Select filled cheeses made with corn, cottonseed, safflower or sunflower seed oils. Avoid coconut or palm oils.

- Cheese with 9 to 11 grams of fat per ounce:

  These cheeses are made from whole milk with added butterfat (milkfat). They are high fat cheeses that contain up to one tablespoon of fat per ounce. One ounce of these cheeses is one high fat meat exchange plus one fat exchange.

Word List

Macadamia: Nut from the tall evergreen silk-oak tree; hard-shelled, shiny round nut with mild delicate flavor. Grown in Hawaii.

Pine nut: Edible sweet flavored nut produced in the pine cone of the nut-bearing pine tree; looks like a large grain of rice. Also called pinon or pignolia.

Pistachio: Seed of a red fruit that has a double shell. The natural color of the seed is green.

Chapter Six
VEGETABLE EXCHANGES

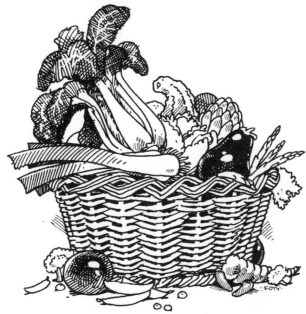

ne half-cup serving of many cooked vegetables is one vegetable exchange. When eaten raw, in amounts less than one cup, vegetables have less than 20 calories and therefore may be considered "free."

One pound of raw vegetables usually yields four half-cup cooked portions. Cooking greens, such as kale and spinach are the exception: one pound yields 8 to 12 half-cup servings, cooked.

Expanded Food List
VEGETABLE

Food value: The following foods contain about 5 grams of carbohydrate, 2 grams of protein and 25 calories. They also contain 2 to 3 grams of fiber. Each equals one vegetable exchange.

Food	Quantity	Exchanges
Artichoke, French/globe	1/2 large cooked, base and soft end of leaves	1 vegetable

Food	Quantity	Exchanges
Artichoke, heart	1/2 heart, cooked	1 vegetable
Artichoke, Jerusalem (Sun choke)	1/4 cup	1 vegetable
Asparagus, cooked	6 large or 8 small spears	1 vegetable
Bamboo shoots, cooked	1 cup	1 vegetable
Common white beans, cooked	1/3 cup	1 vegetable
Yellow snap beans, frozen	1/4 cup	1 vegetable
Bok choy, Chinese chard, white mustard cabbage, cooked	1 cup	1 vegetable
Borscht, beet, cooked	1/2 cup	1 vegetable
Broccoli, cooked	1 large stalk or 2/3 cup	1 vegetable
Carrot juice	1/4 cup (2 fl. oz.)	1 vegetable
Chayote, cooked	1/2 cup or 1/2 medium squash	1 vegetable
Chinese cabbage (Nappa)	2 cup shredded, raw 1 cup shredded, cooked	1 vegetable
Coriander (Chinese parsley)	1 cup	1 vegetable
Collards, boiled	1 cup	1 vegetable
Daikon	1 cup fresh	1 vegetable
Dandelion greens, boiled	1/2 cup	1 vegetable
Eggplant, cooked	3/4 cup	1 vegetable
Jicama, raw	1/2 cup	1 vegetable
Kale, boiled	1/2 cup	1 vegetable
Kohlrabi, raw or cooked	2/3 cup	1 vegetable
Leeks	2 medium	1 vegetable
Mustard greens, cooked	1 cup	1 vegetable
Okra, cooked	8 average pods sliced, 1/2 cup	1 vegetable
Onions, cooked	1/2 cup	1 vegetable

Food	Quantity	Exchanges
Pea pods, **Chinese pea pods** **or snow peas,** cooked	1/2 cup	1 vegetable
Pimento	2 medium or 1/2 cup	1 vegetable
Pumpkin, mashed	1/2 cup	1 vegetable
Rhubarb	1 cup	1 vegetable
Rutabaga, boiled	1/3 cup	1 vegetable
Sauerkraut, canned	1/2 cup	1 vegetable .
Sprouts, **alfalfa, bean, soybean**	1 cup raw, 3/4 cup cooked	1 vegetable
Summer squash, cooked	3/4 cup	1 vegetable
Tomatillos	2	vegetable
Tomatoes, fresh, whole	1 medium	1 vegetable
Tomatoes, cherry	6	1 vegetable
Tomato catsup	2 Tbsp.	1 vegetable
Tomato paste	2 Tbsp. (1 fl. oz.)	1 vegetable
Tomato puree	1/4 cup (2 fl. oz.)	1 vegetable
Tomato sauce	1/3 cup	1 vegetable
Turnips, cooked	1/2 cup	1 vegetable
Turnip greens, canned or cooked	1/2 cup	1 vegetable
V-8 vegetable juice	1/2 cup	1 vegetable
Water chestnuts, **Chinese,** canned	6 whole	1 vegetable
Yard-long beans	1/2 cup	1 vegetable

Word List

Artichokes: Globe artichokes are large unopened buds from a thistle-like plant. You eat them by pulling off the leaves one by one from the cooked artichoke and drawing them between your teeth. The tender heart can be eaten whole. The fuzzy choke at the center should be cut or scooped out and discarded.

Artichoke, Jerusalem (Sun choke): North American native tuber from sunflower plant. Has a sweet, nutty flavor and can be served raw or boiled and used as a potato substitute.

Bok choy: Also known as Chinese chard or white mustard cabbage. It is a green, leafy oriental vegetable with

	slender white stems. It resembles both Swiss chard and celery. Bok choy is a sweet, mild tasting vegetable that can be stir-fried or served raw.
Chayote:	A squash-like vegetable that is light green and pear-shaped. It can be used in any recipe that calls for summer or winter squash.
Chinese cabbage: (Nappa)	A member of the cabbage family, it has a long slender head with long, pale green and white wrinkled leaves. It has a tender texture and a mild, delicate flavor.
Daikon:	A large white radish that can be served raw or pickled. The flavor is slightly hotter than an ordinary radish.
Jicama:	A large, lumpy tuber with dull brown skin. The inside is white, crisp and juicy with water chestnut flavor. Delicious eaten raw.
Kohlrabi:	A member of the cabbage family. Bulbs may be steamed or eaten raw and have a delicate turnip-like taste.
Leeks:	They resemble green onions in shape and flavor but are much larger and milder.
Okra:	Slim, tapered pods that are sometimes nicknamed "lady's fingers." Okra has the power to thicken soups and stews.
Snow peas:	These are sometimes called sugar peas or Chinese peas and have transparent green pods.
Summer squash:	They have soft shells and include: yellow crookneck, straightneck, zucchini (Italian squash), pattypans (scallop or button) and spaghetti squash.
Tomatillos:	Commonly known as ground tomatoes they are small, round-shaped, firm-textured, husk-covered green vegetables. Tart tasting when eaten raw.
Winter squash:	They have hard, firm shells and include: acorn, buttercup, banana, Hubbard and Mediterranean squash. Winter squash is higher in calories than summer squash; a half-cup cooked portion is included on the bread list.
Yard-long beans:	Long and slender in appearance, yard-long beans are related to black-eyed peas and their taste and texture reflect this. They are perfect in long-cooked dishes, adding a chewy-firm, almost meaty texture and taste.

Chapter Seven
FRUIT EXCHANGES

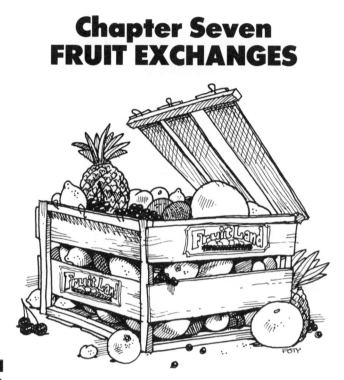

Fruits should be used fresh, dried, canned or frozen without added sugar. Canned fruits may be water packed, artificially sweetened, packed in fruit juice or in their own juice. The serving size for fruit packed in juice includes a small amount of juice. If you wish to use more juice, use a smaller serving of the fruit. Instead of one-half cup use one-third cup fruit with juice for your portion size. Liquid from water packed fruit need not be counted.

Fruits vary in portion size because of their water content. Fruits with a higher water content (strawberries and watermelon) have a larger portion size than fruits with a low water content (bananas and dried fruits). If fruit is dried or canned and you are unsure of the correct portion, use the same amount as you would for fresh fruit. The difference in the fruit is simply the water content. Dried fruit, in the same portion as fresh or raw, may not seem to be as much, but the amount of carbohydrate is the same. If in doubt about portion sizes of fruit, a good rule of thumb is 1/2 cup of fresh fruit or juice or 1/4 cup of dried fruit.

If fruit juices contain sugar, this must be stated on the label. If no mention is made of sugar, you can assume the fruit juice does not contain sugar. Fruit "drinks," "ades" or "punches" contain sugar and should be avoided.

Expanded Food List
FRUIT

Food value: The following foods contain approximately 15 grams of carbohydrate and 60 calories. Fresh, frozen, and dry fruits have about 2 grams of fiber per serving. Fruit juices have very little fiber. Each is one fruit exchange.

Food	Quantity	Exchanges
Berries		
Boysenberries, frozen, unsweetened	1 cup	1 fruit
Elderberries, raw	1/2 cup	1 fruit
Gooseberries	1 cup	1 fruit
Loganberries	3/4 cup	1 fruit
Mulberries, raw	1 cup	1 fruit
Breadfruit	1/8 medium	1 fruit
Carambala (Star fruit)	1½ fruit, 1½ cup cubes	1 fruit
Cherimoya, raw	1/2	1 fruit
Carissa (natal plum)	3/4 cup slices	1 fruit
Casaba melon	1½ cup, cubed, 1 slice, 8″ long × 3″ wide	1 fruit
Cherries		
Fresh, sweet	1/2 cup	1 fruit
Dark sweet	14	1 fruit
Sour red, canned or fresh, water packed	3/4 cup	1 fruit
Citrus salad	3/4 cup	1 fruit
Crabapples, raw	3/4 cup slices	1 fruit
Cranberry sauce	2 Tbsp.	1 fruit
Cranberry-orange relish	2 Tbsp.	1 fruit
Currants, red and white, fresh	1 cup	1 fruit
Fruit cup, fresh	3/4 cup	1 fruit
Fruit cup, frozen, no sugar added	1/2 cup	1 fruit
Fruits for salad	1/2 cup	1 fruit
Groundcherries, raw	1 cup	1 fruit

Food	Quantity	Exchanges
Grapefruit sections	3/4 cup	1 fruit
Granadilla, raw (Passion fruit)	3	1 fruit
Guavas	1 fruit	1 fruit
Homli fruit	1 medium	1 fruit
Java plum, raw	3/4 cup	1 fruit
Kiwi fruit	1½ med. fruit or 1 large	1 fruit
Kumquats, raw	5	1 fruit
Lemon	3 medium	1 fruit
Lime	3 medium	1 fruit
Lychees, litchis	1/2 cup (10)	1 fruit
Loquats, raw	12	1 fruit
Melon balls, frozen	1 cup	1 fruit
Pineapple, canned	1½ slices	1 fruit
Plantains, cooked	1/3 cup	1 fruit
Prickly pears	1½	1 fruit
Quince, raw	1	1 fruit
Raspberries (some sugar added)	1/2 cup	1 fruit
Rhubarb, diced	2 cups	1 fruit
Sapodilla, raw	1/2	1 fruit
Spreadable fruit		
Poiret fruit spread	1 Tbsp.	1 fruit
Polaner all fruit	1 Tbsp.	1 fruit
Tamarinds, raw	12	1 fruit
Tangelos	1	1 fruit
Tropical fruits	1/2 cup	1 fruit
Ugli fruit	3/4 cup	1 fruit
Wild blueberries	1/2 cup	1 fruit
Juices		
Apricot nectar	1/3 cup	1 fruit
Catawba juice	3/4 cup	1 fruit
Cranapple juice, low calorie	1½ cups	1 fruit
Cranberry juice, low calorie	1½ cups	1 fruit
Gatorade	1½ cups (12 fl. oz.)	1 fruit
Hawaiian Punch, low calorie	1 cup	1 fruit

Food	Quantity	Exchanges
Lemon juice	1 cup	1 fruit
Lime juice	1 cup	1 fruit
Peach nectar	1/2 cup	1 fruit
Pear nectar	1/3 cup	1 fruit
Tangerine juice	1/2 cup	1 fruit
Tomato juice	1½ cups	1 fruit
Vegetable juice cocktail	1½ cups	1 fruit

Word List

Carambola (star fruit): When fruit is cut crosswise, it has a star shape. It has a golden yellow color with juicy flesh and crisp texture.

Carob: A long, edible sweet pod that grows on an evergreen tree in the Mediterranean region. It has a flavor like milk chocolate. The pod can be ground and used in baked products. It is also called carob bean, honey bread or locust bean.

Cherimoya: A heart-shaped fruit that is green when ripe and has a skin marked with petal-like indentations. When ripened and chilled, the flesh has a sherbet-like texture. It is also called sweet sop, sherbet fruit, or custard apple.

Guava: A sweet, juicy fruit ranging in color from green to yellow with many small seeds in the center. It is native to Mexico and South America.

Granadilla: (Passion Fruit) It has the size and shape of an egg, a tough purple skin and yellow flesh with black seeds and appears shriveled when ripe and ready to eat.

Homli fruit: A cross between a grapefruit and an orange. It has a greenish skin with orange flesh. The fruit is slightly sweeter than a grapefruit but not as sweet as an orange.

Kiwi fruit:	Brown and elongated with a fuzzy skin. The inside is lime green and similar in texture to the American gooseberry. It is of Chinese origin and now comes from New Zealand or California. It is peeled before eating.
Kumquat:	A small, orange fruit of Chinese origin. It has a very definite citrus flavor. The skin is sweet and the flesh has a tangy flavor. Remove the seeds before eating.
Loquat:	A small, round fruit with yellow-orange skin and pale yellow to orange flesh with black seeds. It comes from a tropical, ornamental evergreen tree. It is very juicy, not too sweet and best when eaten very ripe.
Lychee (Litchi):	An ancient Chinese fruit that is like a strawberry in shape and size. It has a reddish brown, hard skin that is easy to peel. The flesh is white and mild flavored with a single seed and has the consistency of a fresh grape.
Mangoes:	Mangoes may vary in size and shape, depending on the variety and area in which they are grown. They are generally large and oval-shaped with a green to yellow tough skin. Their flesh is orange-yellow and has a rich flavor and spicy aroma. They must be fully ripe before eating.
Persimmon:	It is bright orange in color and has a smooth shiny skin which is removed before eating. It is known as the "apple of the Orient." Persimmons must be very soft before eating or they have a very sour, astringent taste.
Pomegranate:	The name means "apple with many seeds." It is about the size of an orange with a hard skin and deep red color. The inside is filled with edible seeds.
Plantain:	A "cooking banana" with greenish, rough skin. It is an important staple food in tropical countries. Used as a vegetable, the fruit is starchy and is never eaten raw.
Prickly pear:	The fruit of a species of cactus; also called cactus pear. It is yellow to crimson in color, but red when ripe.

Quince:	A very ancient fruit that has hard, tart meat which is not good for eating; good made into a sauce or baked.
Sapote:	It resembles a green apple in appearance; fruit should be firm with greenish to yellow green color. It has a custard-like consistency and flavor and can be eaten fresh.
Tamarind:	A cinnamon-brown, long, flattened pod used in oriental chutneys and curries.
Tangelo:	A citrus fruit with loose skin that is a hybrid of the tangerine. It is the size of a large orange, but the flavor is slightly more tart.
Ugli fruit:	Native to Jamaica, it is about the size of a grapefruit with a disfigured, rough peel. The skin peels off like a tangerine and the pulp is very juicy with an orange-like flavor.

Melons:

Juan canary:	Shaped like a football, bright yellow in color with white flesh tinged with pink around seed cavity. Sweet flavor.
Casaba:	Large round melon with deeply furrowed yellow colored rind and a creamy white flesh. Tastes similar to honeydew, little aroma.
Crenshaw:	Large round melon with pointed stem end. Smooth skin of golden-yellow color with tinges of green. Salmon-colored flesh. Juicy, spicy flavor.
Orange honeydew:	Shaped like a honeydew. Golden tinge to skin with orange flesh.
Persian:	Round melon, similar to cantaloupe. Fine netting over deep green rind. Orange flesh and mildly sweet flavor.
Santa Claus:	Large oblong shaped, similar to small watermelon. Green-gold rind with trace of netting. Yellow-green flesh. Juicy and sweet.
Sharlyn:	Cross between cantaloupe and crenshaw. Color inside is cream to salmon around seed cavity. Netted with greenish background with cream to grey skin. Sweet flavor.

Chapter Eight
MILK EXCHANGES

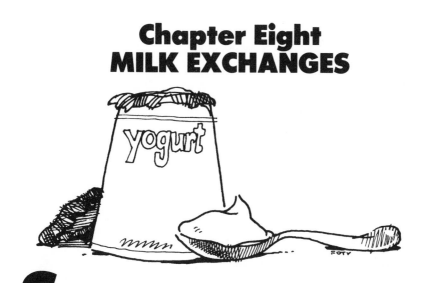

Skim or very lowfat milk is the recommended choice for individuals with diabetes, including children more than two years old. Skim milk is recommended because it contains little or no fat and is low in calories. One percent milk is a good compromise; it contains 3 grams of fat and 100 calories. A low fat diet is important for people with diabetes. Children and individuals who are lean require an adequate amount of calories, but it is not appropriate for a large portion of these calories to be derived from fat.

Plain, lowfat or nonfat unflavored yogurt is an excellent milk substitute. Commercial fruit flavored yogurt is not an ideal milk substitute. Flavored blends of yogurt often rely on imitation flavoring and coloring and contain significant amounts of refined sugar. Some fruit flavored yogurts can actually contain up to 6 teaspoons of sugar. Buy plain yogurt and do the flavoring yourself with fresh or unsweetened fruit or fruit juices. If desired, add Equal® for additional sweetness.

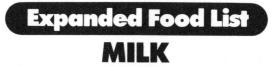

Expanded Food List
MILK

Food value: The following foods contain approximately 12 grams of carbohydrate, 8 grams of protein, a trace of fat and 90 calories. The amount of fat in milk is measured in percent of butterfat. The calories vary, depending on the type of milk. An 8-ounce glass of 2 percent or lowfat milk contains 5 grams of fat and 120 calories. A glass of whole milk has 8 grams of fat and 150 calories.

Food	Quantity	Exchanges
Alba 66 or **Alba 77**	1 envelope	1 skim milk
Cocoa, from mix, artifically sweetened	1 cup	1/2 skim milk
Coconut milk	1/2 cup	1/2 skim milk 6 fat
Eggnog, nonalcoholic	1 cup, 8 fl. oz.	1½ starch/bread 1 skim milk 3 fat
Evaporated milk	1/2 cup	1 whole milk
Evaporated skim milk	1/2 cup	1 skim milk
Filled milk	1 cup	1 whole milk
Goats' milk	1 cup	1 skim milk 2 fat
Soybean milk	1 cup	1/2 med. fat meat 1/2 skim milk
Yogurt, coffee or vanilla flavor	1 cup	1 starch/bread 1 lowfat milk
Weight Watchers nonfat yogurt, plain	1 cup	1 skim milk

The following foods should not be used routinely because they contain a significant amount of sugar. If you choose to use them, use the following exchanges:

Food	Quantity	Exchanges
Cocoa, from mix, water added	1 cup	1 starch/bread 1/2 skim milk
Commercial chocolate milk, made with 1% milk	1 cup	1 starch/bread 1 skim milk
Custard	1/2 cup	1 skim milk 1½ fat
Fruit flavored yogurt	1 cup	2 fruit 1 lowfat milk
Instant breakfast, vanilla with skim milk	1 cup	1½ starch/bread 1 skim milk
Sweet 'n Low nonfat yogurt, all flavors	6 oz.	1½ fruit 3/4 skim milk

Food	Quantity	Exchanges
Weight Watchers Nonfat Yogurt, all flavors	1 cup	1½ fruit 1 milk

Word List

Filled Milk: Milk that contains fats or oils other than milk fat.

Chapter Nine
FAT EXCHANGES

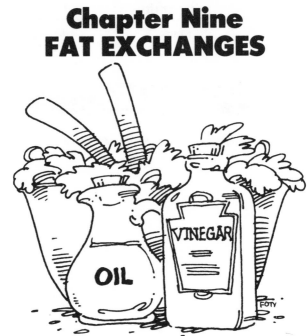

Persons with diabetes should restrict the amount of fat in their diets to approximately 30 percent or less of the total calories. The average American fat intake is 40 to 50 percent of the total calories.

Polyunsaturated fats should be used in place of saturated fats whenever possible. Saturated fats, usually of animal origin, are solid at room temperature. Excessive intake of these fats has been associated with high blood cholesterol levels. Polyunsaturated fats are primarily of vegetable origin and are liquid at room temperature. These fats are thought to help reduce cholesterol levels. Monounsaturated fats are believed to also lower cholesterol levels.

The recommendation to reduce fat, especially saturated fat, can be achieved by:

- limiting meat exchanges to six per day; some women may only need 4 to 5, and persons on meal plans of more than 2,000 calories may be able to have 8.

- using lean meat exchanges whenever possible.

- avoiding high fat meat exchanges such as luncheon meats, frankfurters, sausage and bacon—try to limit these to three times or less per week.

- adding no extra fat in the preparation of foods and cooking away as much fat as possible by baking, broiling or roasting.

- drinking skim milk.
- using low fat or nonfat dairy products such as plain yogurt and skim milk cheeses.
- using margarine instead of butter, but being careful of amounts.
- using vegetable oils whenever possible in baking, cooking and in salad dressing. In most recipes, 3/4 cup liquid vegetable oil may be substituted for 1 cup solid shortening.

Plain yogurt makes an excellent substitute for sour cream or mayonnaise in many recipes. It is lower in calories and fat. Two tablespoons of plain yogurt have approximately 10 to 16 calories; two tablespoons of sour cream, 50 calories; and two tablespoons of mayonnaise, 200 calories.

If a recipe calls for cream, sweet or sour, or mayonnaise, substitute an equal amount of yogurt. To prevent yogurt from separating in cooking, mix one tablespoon of cornstarch with one tablespoon of yogurt. Stir the mixture into one cup of yogurt over medium heat until thickened.

Expanded Food List
FAT

Food value: The following foods contain approximately 5 grams of fat and 45 calories. They are each equivalent to one fat exchange.

Food	Quantity	Exchanges
Unsaturated Fats		
Avocado	1/8 or 2 Tbsp., mashed	1 fat
Blue cheese or Roquefort dressing	2 tsp.	1 fat
Margarines, diet, soft diet, reduced calorie	1 Tbsp.	1 fat
Mayonnaise-type salad dressing, lite	2 Tbsp.	1 fat
Kraft Miracle Whip Light and **Kraft Real Mayonnaise Light**	1 Tbsp.	1 fat
Nuts, chopped	1 Tbsp.	1 fat
Sandwich spread	2 tsp.	1 fat
Shedd's Spread (tub)	2 tsp.	1 fat

Food	Quantity	Exchanges
Shedd's Spread (stick)	1½ tsp.	1 fat
Tahini sesame butter	1 tsp.	1 fat
Tartar sauce	2 tsp.	1 fat
Thousand Island or Russian dressing	2 tsp.	1 fat
Thousand Island, low-calorie	2 Tbsp.	1 fat
Shelled nuts:		
Almonds	7	1 fat
Brazils	2 med.	1 fat
Cashews	4 to 5	1 fat
Filbert	5	1 fat
Macadamia	3	1 fat
Mixed	5 to 6	1 fat
Pecans	5 halves	1 fat
Pinenuts, pignolias	1 Tbsp.	1 fat
Pistachios	15	1 fat
Walnuts	4 halves or 1 Tbsp., chopped	1 fat
Seeds:		
Pumpkin seed kernels	1 Tbsp.	1 fat
Sesame seeds	1 Tbsp.	1 fat
Squash seeds	1 Tbsp.	1 fat
Sunflower seed kernels	1 Tbsp.	1 fat
Saturated Fats		
Anchiote, prepared	1 tsp.	1 fat
Chicken fat	1 tsp.	1 fat
Chitterlings, fried	3/4 oz. (2 Tbsp.)	1 fat
Chicken liver pate, canned	2 Tbsp.	1 fat
Cream cheese, Philadelphia Light	1 oz.	1 fat
Cream cheese dip	1 Tbsp.	1 fat
Cream substitute, non-dairy		
Liquid	2 Tbsp.	1 fat
Powder	4 tsp.	1 fat
French onion dip	2 Tbsp.	1 fat

Food	Quantity	Exchanges
Goose liver pate, canned	1 Tbsp.	1 fat
Gravy	2 Tbsp.	1 fat
Franco-American Gravy— all flavors	1/2 cup	1 fat
Sour cream dips	2 Tbsp.	1 fat
Neufchâtel	3/4 oz.	1 fat
Whipped butter	2 tsp.	1 fat
Whipped toppings, non-dairy		
Frozen	3 Tbsp.	1 fat
From mix	4 Tbsp.	1 fat

Nuts and seeds in larger amounts are counted as 1 medium-fat meat and 2 fat exchanges or as 1 high-fat meat and 1 fat exchange. See the high-fat meat exchange list for portion sizes.

Nondairy creamers contain approximately 20 calories for a 1/2 ounce liquid or 1½ teaspoons powdered portion. One portion may be considered "free" or equivalent to 1/2 fat exchange. However, these products are usually made from palm or coconut oils or other hydrogenated vegetable oils, which are saturated fats and therefore are not recommended for use. Instead try using a teaspoon of instant nonfat dry milk. This contains only 10 calories per teaspoon and is considered a "free" food. When using milk in hot beverages, allow the beverage to cool for a few minutes so the powder will dissolve without a curdled appearance.

Chapter Ten
FREE FOODS

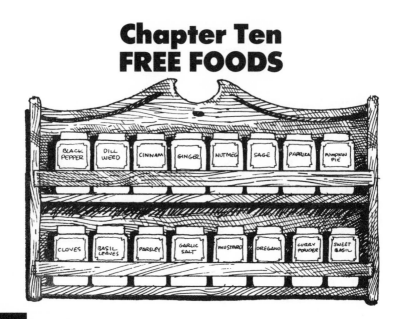

Free foods are those with relatively few calories, less than 20 per serving. Limit free foods to a total of 50 to 60 calories per day, divided between meals and snacks.

Expanded Food List
FREE FOODS

Food value: The following foods are noncaloric or negligible in calories (less than 20 calories per serving). Maximum serving size is noted when the amount should be limited.

Food	Quantity	Exchanges
A-1 sauce or steak sauce	1 Tbsp.	free
Beverage or drink mixes		
Sugar free		free
Iced tea mix with Nutrasweet®		free
Butter Buds	1 oz. liquid	free
Bouillon or broths (dry)	1 packet, 1 tsp., or 1 cube	free
Bouillon or broths (canned)	3/4 cup	free
Catsup, tomato	1 Tbsp.	free

Food	Quantity	Exchanges
Cocoa, dry unsweetened	1 Tbsp.	free
Coffee whiteners, powdered	1 tsp.	free
Chili sauce	1 Tbsp.	free
Chocolate topping, reduced calorie or low calorie	1 Tbsp.	free
Club soda, carbonated water (not tonic water or quinine water)		free
Comet cones or cups	1	free
Cool Whip	1 Tbsp.	free
Cranberries, cooked without sugar	1/2 cup	free
Diet, "low carbohydrate" "sugar-free" hard candies	Amount not to exceed 20 calories	free
Low-calorie or reduced-calorie syrup	Amount not to exceed 20 calories	free
Dill pickle	1	free
Dream Whip	1 Tbsp.	free
D-Zerta		
Gelatin, unflavored plain		free
Gelatin dessert, artificially sweetened		free
Gum, sugar-free		free
Jalapeno bean dip	2 Tbsp.	free
Jams and jellies, artificially sweetened	Amount not to exceed 20 calories	free
Low sugar	2 tsp.	free
Horseradish	3 Tbsp.	free
Kool-Aid, unsweetened		free
Lemon or orange rind		free
Milk flavorings		
Nestlé, Ovaltine	1 heaping tsp. or 2½ level tsp.	free
Swiss Miss Sugar Free, all flavors	1 heaping tsp. or 2½ level tsp.	free
Mustard, prepared	1 Tbsp.	free

Food	Quantity	Exchanges
Onion		free
Pickle relish		free
Pimiento		free
Postum, instant powder	2 tsp.	free
Salad dressing, low calorie	Amount not to exceed 20 calories	free
Sauerkraut juice	1 cup	free
Sour Slim or sour half and half	1 Tbsp.	free
Soy sauce	1 Tbsp.	free
Sugar substitutes		free
Tabasco sauce	1 Tbsp.	free
Taco hot sauce	1 Tbsp.	free
Tomato paste	1 Tbsp.	free
Tomato puree	1 Tbsp.	free
Vinegar		free
Weight Watchers gravies, dressings, dip	1/4 cup	free
Worcestershire sauce	1 Tbsp.	free
Yeast, brewer's	2 tsp.	free
Yogurt, plain	2 Tbsp.	free
Vegetable pan spray		free
Whipped topping, low calorie	2 Tbsp.	free

Spices are also free foods. The following seasonings may be used without including them as exchanges in your meal plan.

Allspice	Cumin	Paprika
Angostura bitters	Curry	Parsley
Anise	Dill	Pepper
Basil	Extracts, vanilla, etc.	Poppy seed
Bay leaf	Garlic	Poultry seasoning
Caraway	Ginger root	Rosemary
Cardamon	Mace	Saffron
Celery salt or seed	Marjoram	Sage
Chervil	Mint	Sesame seed
Chili powder	Monosodium glutamate	Tenderizers
Chives	Mustard, dry	Thyme
Cinnamon	Nutmeg	
Cloves	Oregano	

Chapter Eleven
COMBINATION FOODS

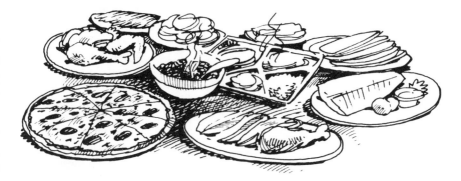

Many foods are a combination of foods from several of the exchange lists. Some common ones are listed below. They will, of course, vary depending on the ingredients, and these are average values. If in doubt, count one cup of a casserole or hot dish as 2 starch/bread exchanges, 2 medium-fat meats, and 0-1 fat exchange. (Looks like a sandwich, doesn't it?) This will be a good rule-of-thumb and will allow you to add variety to your meal planning.

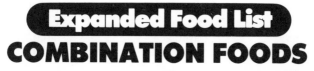

COMBINATION FOODS

Food	Quantity	Exchanges
Main Dishes		
Beans and Ham	1 cup	3 starch/bread 2 lean meat
Beef, chicken, turkey pie (homemade)	1 cup	3 starch/bread 2 med. fat meat 4 fat
Beef Vegetable Stew (homemade)	1 cup	2 starch/bread 2 med. fat meat
Creamed Chipped Beef	1/2 cup	2 med. fat meat 1 fat

Food	Quantity	Exchanges
Chicken A La King (homemade)	1 cup	1 starch/bread 2 med. fat meat 3 fat
Chicken and noodles (homemade)	1 cup	2 starch/bread 2 med. fat meat 1 fat
Chili Con Carne with Beans (homemade)	1 cup	2 starch/bread 2 med. fat meat 1 fat
Chow Mein	1½ cups	1 starch/bread 2 med. fat meat 1 vegetable
Beef Chop Suey (homemade)	1 cup	1 starch/bread 3 med. fat meat
Corned Beef Hash (homemade)	1 cup	2 starch/bread 2 med. fat meat
French Toast	2 slices	2 starch/bread 1 med. fat meat 1 fat
Ham and lima bean casserole (homemade)	1 cup	3 starch/bread 3 med. fat meat
Pizza, cheese (homemade)	1 small slice	1 starch/bread 1 med. fat meat
Pizza—13½ oz.	1/4 pizza	1 starch/bread 1 med. fat meat 1 vegetable 1 fat
Stuffed Pepper	1 average	2 starch/bread 2 med. fat meat
Potato Pancakes	2 average (3-inch diameter)	1 starch/bread 1 fat
Spanish Rice	1 cup	3 starch/bread 1 fat
Souffle, cheese	4 oz.	1/2 starch/bread 2 med. fat meat 2 fat
Spaghetti and Meat Balls with Tomato Sauce (homemade)	1 cup	2 starch/bread 2 med. fat meat 1 vegetable
Veal Scallopini	6 oz.	4 med. fat meat 1 vegetable
Welsh Rarebit	1 cup	1 starch/bread 2 med. fat meat 4 fat

Food	Quantity	Exchanges
Salads		
Caesar salad	1 serving	2 vegetable 6 fat
Chef's salad (mixed greens, 3 Tbsp. regular dressing, 1 oz. cheese, chicken and ham)	1 serving	1 starch/bread **or** 3 vegetable 3 med. fat meat 2 fat
Chicken salad	1/2 cup	2 med. fat meat 2 fat
Coleslaw	1/2 cup	1 vegetable 2 fat
Egg salad	1/2 cup	1 med. fat meat 4 fat
Potato salad (homemade)	1/2 cup	1 starch/bread 1-2 fat
Tuna salad	1/2 cup	2 med. fat meat 1 fat
Waldorf salad	1/2 cup	1/2 fruit 3 fat
Sandwiches		
Bacon, lettuce, tomato, mayonnaise	1 sandwich	2 starch/bread 3 fat
Chicken, lettuce, mayonnaise	1 sandwich	2 starch/bread 2 med. fat meat 1 fat
Chicken salad	1 sandwich	2 starch/bread 2 med. fat meat
Club sandwich (bacon, chicken, tomato, lettuce and mayonnaise on 3 slices bread)	1 sandwich	3 starch/bread 4 med. fat meat 1 fat
Corned beef	1 sandwich	2 starch/bread 3 med. fat meat
Egg salad	1 sandwich	2 starch/bread 1 med. fat meat 1 fat
Grilled cheese	1 sandwich	2 starch/bread 2 med. fat meat 2 fat
Ham salad	1 sandwich	2 starch/bread 1 med. fat meat 2 fat

53

Food	Quantity	Exchanges
Hot dog (frank) in roll	1	1½ starch/bread 1 high fat meat 2 fat
Liverwurst	1 sandwich	2 starch/bread 1 high fat meat 2 fat
Meat loaf	1 sandwich	2 starch/bread 3 med. fat meat
Peanut butter	1 sandwich	2 starch/bread 1 high fat meat 2 fat
Roast beef and gravy	1 sandwich	2 starch/bread 2 med. fat meat 3 fat
Roast pork and gravy	1 sandwich	2 starch/bread 2 med. fat meat 4 fat
Submarine sandwich or Hoagie	1 large	4 starch/bread 4 med. fat meat 1 fat
Tuna salad	1 sandwich	2 starch/bread 1 med. fat meat 2 fat

Chapter Twelve
SPECIAL OCCASION FOODS

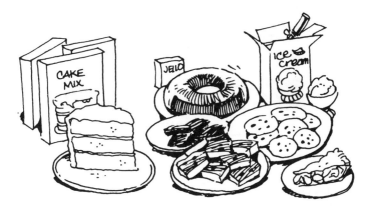

Some foods can occasionally be used as starch/bread or fruit exchanges despite the fact they contain refined sugars. Because they contain refined sugars (and often are high in fat as well), their use should be restricted. If you choose to use these foods, the most appropriate times are with a meal or a snack before exercise. At meals the other foods seem to slow absorption of sugars, and exercise can also help to lower blood glucose levels. See chapter 24 for exercise guidelines.

Dietitians are frequently asked, "What is occasional?" "How often should individuals substitute these foods in their meal plan?" These are difficult questions because what may be "occasional" for one family or person can be "frequent" for another. Perhaps the best advice is that everyone, including individuals with diabetes, can benefit from avoiding foods high in sugar. These foods are often high in fat and calories as well and provide only calories without any other important nutrients—what we call "empty calories."

The fact that an individual has diabetes may have less to do with metabolism of sugar than we believed in the past. No one can eat large amounts of these foods and stay thin, just as individuals with diabetes cannot eat large amounts of these foods without elevating their blood glucose. However, if it is your choice to use these foods, you need to know how to do so correctly—how to substitute correctly in your meal plan. You will notice the portion sizes are very small, since these foods often are concentrated sources of carbohydrates and fat.

Remember the goal of meal planning is to help you keep your blood glucose and fats as normal and optimal as possible—as well as to control your weight. Checking your blood glucose one or two hours after a meal may help you know how these foods are affecting your blood glucose values. Having your doctor check your glycosylated hemoglobin values (a test that helps evaluate your overall blood glucose during the past four to six weeks) and blood fats (cholesterol and triglycerides) will also help you know how well you are meeting your nutritional goals.

Special Foods

Food	Quantity	Exchanges
Apple Brown Betty	1/2 cup	2 starch/bread 1 fruit 1 fat
Baked apples (unpared, average 2 Tbsp. sugar)	1/2 average	1½ fruit
Brownies, chocolate	1 average, 2″ by 2″	1 starch/bread 1 fat
Cakes		
Angel food cake	1 slice, 1/12th cake	2 starch/bread
Commercial cake mix (chocolate, white, yellow, lemon, etc., from mix)	1/12 cake	2 starch/bread 2 fat
Gingerbread, from mix	1/9 cake	2 starch/bread 1 fat
Poundcake, homemade	1 slice (1 oz.)	1 starch/bread 2 fat
Spice cake, from mix	1/12 cake	2 starch/bread 1 fat
Carrot cake, from mix	1/12 cake	2 starch/bread 2 fat
Shortcake	1 average	1 starch/bread
Cookies		
In general, 3″ diameter	1	1 starch/bread
1¾″ diameter	2	1 starch/bread
Animal	12 small	1 starch/bread
Chocolate chip, 1¾″ diameter	2	1 starch/bread 1 fat

Food	Quantity	Exchanges
Fig bar	2	1½ starch/bread
Gingersnaps	5 small	1 starch/bread
Fortune cookies	2	1 starch/bread
Lady fingers	1 large or 2 small	1 starch/bread
Lorna Doone shortbread	3	1 starch/bread 1 fat
Oatmeal raisin	2	1 starch/bread 1 fat
Oreo creme sandwich (not with extra filling)	2	1 starch/bread 1 fat
Social tea biscuits, plain	4	1 starch/bread
Sugar cookies	2 average	2 starch/bread 1 fat
Vanilla wafers	6 small	1 starch/bread
Chocolate syrup	2 Tbsp.	1 starch/bread
Cream puff shell	1	1 starch/bread 2 fat
Cupcake, no icing, from mix	1 average	1 starch/bread
Custard, baked	1/2 cup	1 starch/bread 1 med. fat meat
Doughnuts, plain, cake type or raised	1 average	1 starch/bread 1 fat
Frozen desserts		
Drumstick	1 average	1½ starch/bread 2 fat
Fudgesicle	1 average	1 starch/bread
Ice cream, all flavors	1/2 cup	1 starch/bread 2 fat
Ice cream bars, vanilla, chocolate coated	1 average	1 starch/bread 2 fat
Ice cream sandwich	1 average	2 starch/bread 1 fat
Ice cream, soft serve	1/2 cup	1 starch/bread 2 fat
Ice milk, all flavors	1/2 cup	1 starch/bread 1 fat
Ice milk, soft serve	1/2 cup	1 starch/bread 1 fat
Milkshake, chocolate or vanilla, thick	8 fl. oz.	3 starch/bread 1 fat

Food	Quantity	Exchanges
Popsicle	1 bar	1 starch/bread or 1 fruit
Popsicle, twin pop	1 bar	1½ fruit
Sherbet, all flavors	1/4 cup	1 starch/bread
Sorbet	1/4 cup	1 starch/bread
Yogurt, frozen, fruit varieties	8 oz.	2 starch/bread 1/2 milk
Frozen fruit/juice bar	1 bar	1 fruit
Fruit rolls or roll-ups	1 roll	1 fruit
Fruit bar	1 bar	1½ fruit
Gelatin dessert, all flavors	1/2 cup	1 starch/bread **or** 1 fruit
Granola bar	1 bar	1 starch/bread 1/2 fat
Ice cream cone **(cone only)**	1	1/2 starch/bread
Malt powder, plain, dry	2 Tbsp.	1 starch/bread
Pastry	1/6 9″ pie crust	1 starch/bread 2 fat
Patty shell	1 shell	1 starch/bread 4 fat
Pie crust, **graham cracker crumb**	1/6 9″pie crust	1 starch/bread 2 fat
Pudding		
Vanilla or chocolate, instant, from mix	1/2 cup	2 starch/bread 1 fat
Rice pudding	1/2 cup	2 starch/bread 1 fat
Tapioca	1/2 cup	2 starch/bread 1 fat
Pudding pops	1 pop	1 starch/bread 1/2 fat
Syrups, Lite	2 Tbsp.	1 starch/bread

The following foods in the amounts listed also contain 15 grams of carbohydrate and are the equivalent of one fruit exchange. They are not recommended for use because they contain significant amounts of refined sugars. However, you may find them convenient to use to treat insulin reactions or to prevent hypoglycemia during exercise.

Food	Quantity	Exchanges
Butterscotch balls	3	1 fruit
Carbonated beverages, regular	3/4 cup (6 oz.)	1 fruit
Corn syrup or honey	3 tsp.	1 fruit
Gelatin, sweetened, prepared	1/2 cup	1 fruit
Granulated sugar	4 tsp.	1 fruit
Gum drops	18 average	1 fruit
Hard candy	3 average	1 fruit
Honey	1 Tbsp.	1 fruit
Jelly beans	9	1 fruit
Lemon drops	8	1 fruit
LifeSavers	8	1 fruit
Marshmallows	3 large	1 fruit
Maple syrup	1/4 cup	4 fruit

Part II

EXCHANGES FOR
SPECIAL OCCASIONS

Chapter Thirteen
ADDING FIBER TO YOUR DIET

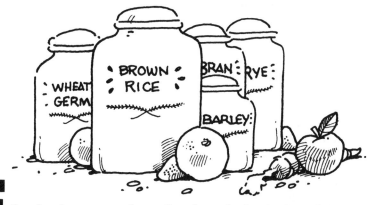

Fiber has been part of our diet since the beginning of time. Your grandmother may have called it "roughage" or "bulk." Although not new, its importance has been recognized only since the 1960s. In the '80s we have gone from calling fiber a "cure-all" for all health problems, including diabetes, back to more moderate recommendations that all Americans should try to gradually increase the fiber content in their diet.

What is fiber?

A complex carbohydrate, fiber is the structural part (or cell walls) of fruits, vegetables, and grains that cannot be digested or broken down in the human digestive tract and absorbed into the bloodstream. It does not supply nutrients. There are two types of dietary fiber—insoluble and soluble—and each has specific benefits.

Insoluble fiber does not dissolve in water. This fiber gives plants structure. Its major components are celluloses (structural material in cell walls of plants), hemicelluloses (also found in plants but less complex than cellulose), and lignin (non-carbohydrate product that, with cellulose, forms the wood cell wall of plants). Common sources of insoluble fibers are wheat and corn bran, whole grains, some vegetables, and nuts. Insoluble fibers are able to retain large amounts of water, thus increasing the volume of the stool and making it pass faster through the intestinal tract. Therefore, these fibers help prevent and treat constipation and diverticulosis, and may even help to prevent certain types of cancer, such as cancer of the colon and rectum.

Soluble fibers form a gel in water and include gums (with a gel-like texture, found in oats and legumes) mucilages (a gelatinous substance found in seeds), and pectin (found in fruits, especially citrus fruits and apples). Soluble fibers can bind bile salts, cholesterol and other sterols, thus reducing their absorption from the intestinal tract. These fibers have been found to lower cholesterol and may offer some improvement in carbohydrate metabolism in people with diabetes. It is important to include foods that contain both soluble and insoluble fibers, because both are important for health and well-being.

Why eat fiber?

Interest in fiber began in the 1960s when an English doctor, Denis Burkitt, reported on rural Africans whose diets were high in fiber. They had a much lower incidence of cancer of the large intestine than did Americans or Europeans eating a low fiber diet. Diverticulitis (small pouches) of the colon walls, appendicitis, gallstones, varicose veins, hemorrhoids, some forms of coronary heart disease, and diabetes all occurred with much less frequency in the Africans who consumed 50 to 150 grams of dietary fiber per day compared to the Americans' 10 to 20 grams per day.

These and other epidemiological studies—studies of diseases as they appear in populations of people—along with animal research have provided evidence of the benefits of fiber. None of the evidence can be regarded as conclusive, however. One reason is that the epidemiological evidence is subject to many possible interpretations. There are also many differences between population groups, not only in diet, but in other aspects of life as well. In addition, people who eat more fiber tend to also eat less fat. High fat and high calorie diets as well as low fiber diets have been shown to increase risk of some diseases. The animal studies are suggestive rather than conclusive. And finally, results of the studies have been mixed.

Nevertheless, research indicates a relationship between a high fiber diet and good health. Consequently, Americans have been encouraged by health and government agencies to consume less fat while increasing complex carbohydrate and fiber. Fiber is also thought to be beneficial for certain health problems:

Gastrointestinal problems.—Fiber increases stool bulk and size because of water-holding capacity and therefore accelerates intestinal transit time. Wheat bran is widely used to treat constipation. Constipation can contribute to hemorrhoids, varicose veins, and diverticular disease of the colon.

Cancer.—If there are carcinogens (cancer-causing agents) in food, fiber speeds up transit time of stools through the digestive system, thus reducing exposure time to these carcinogens. Fiber may also be able to bind a carcinogen, thus making it unavailable. Both the National Cancer Institute and the American Cancer Society have recommended low fat diets generous in dietary fiber to reduce risk of colon, rectal, breast, and prostate cancer.

Obesity.—Diets high in fiber can promote long-term weight loss and maintenance because foods containing fiber are typically low in fat and generally take longer to chew, thus slowing food intake. They also slow the emptying of foods from the stomach, contributing to the feeling of fullness, and since fiber is nondigestible it contributes practically no calories.

Coronary Heart Disease.—Diets rich in soluble fiber have been shown to lower blood cholesterol and raise high-density lipoprotein (HDL or "good" cholesterol), which protects against heart disease. Fiber may also maintain or lower triglycerides.

Hypertension.—Some evidence is also beginning to suggest that dietary fiber may lower blood pressure.

Diabetes.—High-fiber diets also offer health benefits for persons with diabetes. Generous fiber intake may be able to help lower blood glucose and insulin levels and improve glycemic control. High fiber intake also lowers serum cholesterol and triglyceride levels in persons with diabetes. Because diabetes can accelerate heart disease, maintaining normal lipid (fat) levels is a primary goal of diabetes management.

Although some studies have suggested that dietary fiber can be effective in controlling blood glucose and cholesterol levels, a recent National Institutes of Health Concensus Panel on Noninsulin-Dependent Diabetes found the results of these studies to be inconclusive. Nevertheless, people with diabetes should include fiber in their diets for the same health reasons that all Americans should.

How much fiber should you consume?

It is currently estimated that the average dietary fiber intake is between 10 to 30 grams per day, with men averaging 19 grams per day and women 13 grams. For most individuals, a practical goal would be to estimate current fiber intake and gradually increase it, with the goal of doubling the intake. An intake of up to 40 grams of fiber per day or approximately 25 grams of fiber for every 1,000 calories you eat appears to be beneficial.

It is important not to go overboard with fiber; too much fiber can inhibit the absorption of important vitamins and minerals in foods and can cause gas, diarrhea, and bloating. These side effects of fiber can make high levels unacceptable. The level of maximum benefit has not been determined, but a maximum intake of 50 grams per day seems reasonable. Children may also benefit from an increase in the fiber content of their diets, but younger children may not tolerate large amounts of fiber.

There is insufficient evidence on the long-term safety of high-fiber supplements. Fiber supplementation appears to be of benefit only if given with a high carbohydrate diet. Use fiber supplements only under your physician's advice. It is generally recommended that foods should be selected with moderate to high amounts of dietary fiber from a wide variety of foods, instead of from supplements. These foods include legumes, lentils, roots, tubers, green leafy vegetables, all types of whole-grain cereals (e.g. wheat, barley, oats, corn and rye) breads and pasta, bran, fruits, nuts, and seeds. Bran cereal is an especially concentrated source of fiber.

An added benefit of eating a high fiber diet is that, although fiber is classified as a carbohydrate and therefore is included on food labels as total carbohydrate, it is nondigestible and contributes virtually no calories. The grams of carbohydrate from fiber are not included in the calorie calculation.

The following guidelines will help you to add fiber to your diet.

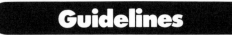

Guidelines

- **Increase your fiber intake slowly.** Digestive discomfort from intestinal gas may occur when fiber intake is increased. Generally, this is only a temporary problem and will subside as the body adjusts to a higher fiber diet. This problem can be minimized by increasing fiber intake gradually. Start with small servings and increase portions gradually.

- **Eat a variety of fiber-rich foods in reasonable amounts.** Increase your intake of whole grain breads and cereals. Cereals can be excellent sources of fiber and make good choices for breakfast. Include more fruits and vegetables in your diet. Your fiber source should be food, not fiber supplements. Fiber supplements usually do not contain large amounts of dietary fiber, nor do they have all the other nutrients that accompany fiber in foods.

- **Go for carbohydrates packaged in their natural fibrous coatings.** Examples are brown rice instead of white rice; whole-grain flour instead of white flour; peelings on fruits and vegetables; whole fruits instead of juice; baked potato with skin instead of mashed potatoes.

- **Try to drink eight glasses of water a day.** Since fiber attracts water, it is important to drink enough liquids when you add fiber to your diet. This keeps everything moving through the intestinal tract and helps prevent constipation.

- **Buy whole-grain bread** made from stone ground flour, 100% whole wheat, or other whole grain flour. "Brown breads" contain little or no whole grain, just molasses for coloring. If the label says "wheat flour" remember almost all flours are made from wheat, and this phrase usually refers to bleached white flour. When buying breads and cereals, "whole grain," "whole wheat," or "whole oats" should be first on the ingredient list. You get the most nutrients and the best flavor from stone-ground whole-wheat flour. Second best is ordinary whole-wheat flour. You can also buy whole-wheat pastry flour.

- **Use raw fruits** with skins (such as apples), membranes (such as oranges) or seeds (such as strawberries) instead of fruit juices. Include more raw and slightly cooked vegetables such as corn, peas, beans, legumes, and potatoes with the skin. The stems and leaves of salad greens and broccoli are also fibrous. Don't throw away these good fiber sources.

- **Watch those calories.** If you add extra calories by adding high-fiber foods to your daily eating instead of substituting them for some food choices, you will probably gain weight as well as causing your blood glucose to rise. To save calories, trim your intake of high-fat, high-calorie foods such as cream, gravies, sauces, and salad dressings. Eat breads and vegetables without margarine or butter; use noncaloric products (such as Pam) for "greasing" pans; use nonstick pans.

- **Choose lean meats** and do not exceed the recommended amount (usually 4 to 6 ounces per day).

- **Limit fat and oil.**

Now you know the basics of high fiber eating, but how do you plan meals? The 1986 revision of *Exchange Lists for Meal Planning* can help you. A symbol for fiber has been placed next to foods that contain 3 grams or more of dietary fiber per serving. Servings from the fruit list, vegetable list and the whole-grain breads and cracker list have 2 grams of dietary fiber. To help you choose foods high in fiber the following is a general guide giving you average fiber values for foods on the exchange list.

LIST 1. STARCH/BREAD

NUTRIENT VALUES: 15 grams carbohydrates; 3 grams protein; trace fat; 80 calories

Cereals:

FIBER: One serving of cereal averages 2 to 3 grams of fiber and 1 starch/bread exchange unless otherwise specified.

Good Choices	Quantity
*All Bran or Bran Buds	1/3 cup
*100% Bran	1/3 cup
**Fiber One	1/2 cup
Bran Chex	1/2 cup
Bran Flakes, 40%	1/2 cup
Bran Flakes with Raisins	1/2 cup
Corn Bran	1/2 cup
Cracklin' Oat Bran	1/2 cup
Most	1/2 cup
Nutri Grain	1/2 cup
Oatflakes, fortified	1/2 cup
Shredded Wheat	1/2 cup or 1 large biscuit
Total	1/2 cup
Wheaties	3/4 cup
Cooked Cereals	
Oats (oatmeal)	1/2 cup
Oat Bran	1/2 cup
Ralstons (whole wheat)	1/2 cup

*8 grams fiber
**12 grams fiber

Grains and Breads:

FIBER: One serving of bread or grains average 2 grams of fiber and 1 starch/bread exchange.

Good Choices	Quantity
Barley, cooked	1/3 cup
Buckwheat, Kasha, cooked	1/3 cup
Bulgur, cooked	1/2 cup
Couscous, cooked	1/3 cup
Cornmeal	2½ Tbsp.
Graham crackers	3 squares
Grits, cooked	1/2 cup
Muffins; bran, oat, corn	1/2 muffin
Popcorn	3 cups
Rice, brown or wild, cooked	1/3 cup
Ry Krisp	3 triple crackers or 4 squares

Rye, pumpernickel, whole wheat, whole meal or cracked wheat bread	1 slice
Tortilla, corn	1
Wheat bran (no calories)	1½ Tbsp.
Whole-wheat crackers	4 to 5
Whole-wheat roll	1
Wheat germ	3 Tbsp.
Miller's bran	1/4 cup
Wheat bran	1/2 cup

Starchy Vegetables:

FIBER: One serving of starchy vegetables averages 3 grams of fiber and 1 starch/bread exchange.

Good Choices	Quantity
Corn, cooked	1/2 cup
Corn on cob	1 small
Lima beans	1/2 cup
Peas, garden	1/2 cup
Plantain	1/2 cup
Potato, baked with skin	1 small
Squash, winter (acorn)	1 cup
Sweet potatoes, cooked	1/3 cup

Dried Beans, Peas, Lentils:

FIBER: One serving of legumes averages 5 grams of fiber and 1 starch/bread exchange.

Good Choices	Quantity
Cooked or canned dried beans (kidney, navy, pinto, etc.), dried peas, lentils	1/3 cup
Canned baked beans	1/4 cup

Each 1/3 cup serving contains about 5 grams of protein and 13 grams of carbohydrate. If used as 1 starch/bread exchange it is not necessary to compensate for the extra protein. When consuming larger portions (1 cup), count as 2 starch/bread and 1 lean meat exchange.

LIST 2. MEAT AND SUBSTITUTES

NUTRIENT VALUES: 5 grams protein; 8 grams fat; 100 calories. Meat and meat products do not contain any significant amount of fiber. The exception is all varieties of nuts as well as pumpkin, sesame, and sunflower seeds. However, each 1/2 ounce serving also contains 100 calories.

FIBER: One serving (1/2 oz. nuts or seeds) averages 2 grams of fiber and 1 high fat meat exchange.

Good Choices	Quantity
Nuts or seeds	1/2 oz. (2 Tbsp.)
Peanut butter	1 Tbsp.

LIST 3. VEGETABLES

NUTRIENT VALUES: 5 grams carbohydrates; 2 grams protein; 25 calories

FIBER: One serving (1/2 cup cooked or 1 cup raw) averages 2 grams fiber.

LIST 4. FRUITS

NUTRIENTS: 15 grams carbohydrates; 60 calories

FIBER: One serving (1/2 cup or 1 medium fruit) averages 2 grams fiber.

LIST 5. MILK

Milk products do not have fiber.

LIST 6. FATS

Fat products do not have fiber.

Sample Menu

HIGH FIBER, HIGH CARBOHYDRATE 1500 CALORIES

	Meal Plan (Exchanges)	Menu (Foods)	Fiber (Grams)
Breakfast:	2 Starch/Bread	2/3 cup All Bran	16
	1 Fruit	1 medium orange	2
	1/2 Skim Milk	1/2 cup skim milk	0
Snack:	1 Fruit	1 apple	2
Lunch:	2 Starch/Bread	2 slices whole-wheat bread	4
	1 Meat	1 oz. slice turkey	0
	1 Vegetable	2 cups lettuce with reduced calorie dressing	2
	1 Fruit	15 grapes	2
	1 Skim Milk	1 cup skim milk	0
	1 Fat	1 tsp. margarine	0
Snack:	1 Starch/Bread	4 squares Ry Krisp	2
Dinner:	1 Starch/Bread	1/3 cup brown rice	2
	1 Starch/Bread	1 whole-wheat roll	2
	3 Meat	3 oz. broiled fish	0
	1 Vegetable	1 cup broccoli	2
	1 Vegetable	2 cups lettuce with reduced-calorie dressing	2
	1 Fruit	1/3 cup pineapple chunks	2
	1 Fat	1 tsp. margarine	0
Evening Snack:	1 Starch/Bread	3 cups popcorn, no butter	2
	1/2 Skim Milk	1/2 cup skim milk	0
Totals:	1500 calories	220 gms. CHO (61%) 75 gms. protein (21%) 30 gms. fat (18%) 42 gms. of FIBER	

Chapter Fourteen
IF YOU CHOOSE TO BE VEGETARIAN

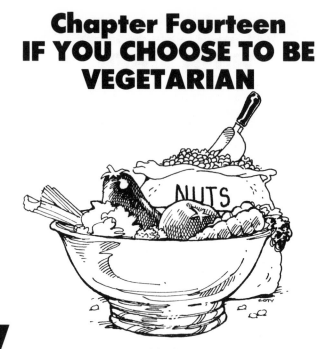

Vegetarian eating is possible for individuals with diabetes. People may choose such a diet for economic, religious, ethnic or health reasons. Whatever your motivation, if you have chosen or are considering a vegetarian way of eating, you will find this section helpful.

The first step is to work with a dietitian to design a vegetarian meal plan suited to your lifestyle. Vegetarians must necessarily use more whole grain products and legumes than nonvegetarians. Whole grains and legumes are excellent sources of vitamins, minerals, and protein. They also are excellent sources of fiber.

There are three different types of vegetarian diets. A lacto-ovo-vegetarian diet includes plant foods, eggs and dairy products but excludes meat, poultry and fish. A lacto-vegetarian diet includes plant foods and dairy products but excludes meat, poultry, fish and eggs. A strict vegetarian diet includes only foods from plant sources and excludes all foods of animal origin. Protein in a lacto-ovo-vegetarian diet is supplied mainly from dairy products, eggs and legumes. In the strict vegetarian diet, legumes, grains, soymilk and meat analogs (meat substitutes, usually made from soy products) supply most of the protein.

Both the quality and quantity of the protein we eat is important. Beans, peas and lentils are a primary source of protein in much of the world. They are considered "incomplete" proteins, meaning that they lack or are low in certain amino acids needed by the body to synthesize protein.

Amino acids are the building blocks of protein. There are nine amino acids that cannot be made by the body and must come from food. These are called essential amino acids. However, different plant proteins can be combined so the essential amino acid missing in one is supplied by the second plant source. Soybeans are the exception. They are a complete protein by themselves.

These combinations supply complete proteins. Combine the protein source at the top with any listed beneath it:

Rice	**Wheat**	**Legumes**
Wheat	Legumes	Corn
Legumes	Soybeans and	Rice
Nuts and seeds	peanuts	Wheat
	Soybeans and seeds	Nuts and seeds
	Rice and soybeans	Barley
		Oats

The amino acids in milk products and eggs also complement plant proteins.

A one-cup serving of cooked legumes with a complementary plant protein or small amount of animal protein (milk, cheese, eggs) replaces a three-ounce portion of meat, fish or poultry. Foods that originate from plants contain no saturated fat or cholesterol, an added benefit.

Vegetable proteins have been prepared commercially to simulate many meat products. Included in this list are steaks, chops, wieners, hamburger-style products and dehydrated burger granules. These meat analogs can add interest and variety to the lacto-ovo-vegetarian diet.

One caution: vitamin B_{12} is an essential vitamin needed to prevent anemia. It is present only in animal food products. Strict vegetarians will need to select fortified cereals, soymilk or meat analogs or take a B_{12} supplement. In the lacto-ovo-vegetarian diet, eggs, cheese, milk or yogurt supply vitamin B_{12}.

Expanded Exchanges
VEGETARIAN DIET

Food	Quantity	Exchanges
Starch/Bread		
Arabic bread, Syrian bread	1/2 of a 2½ oz. loaf	1 starch/bread
Barley, cooked	1/3 cup	1 starch/bread
Brown rice, cooked	1/3 cup	1 starch/bread
Buckwheat flour (dark or light)	3 Tbsp.	1 starch/bread
Buckwheat, Kasha, groats, cooked	1/3 cup	1 starch/bread
Bulgur, cooked	1/2 cup	1 starch/bread
Bulgur, dry	2 Tbsp.	1 starch/bread
Couscous	1/3 cup	1 starch/bread
Millet, cooked	2/3 cup	1 starch/bread
Miso	3 Tbsp.	1 starch/bread
Oats, cooked	1/2 cup	1 starch/bread
Pocket bread or pita, 4½" diameter	1	1 starch/bread
Pocket bread or pita, 6" diameter	1	1 starch/bread
Rye flour	3 Tbsp.	1 starch/bread
Soybean flour, full fat	1/2 cup	1 starch/bread 2 med. fat meat
Soybean flour, low fat	1/2 cup	1 starch/bread 3 lean meat
Wheat berries, cooked	2/3 cup	1 starch/bread
Wild rice, cooked	1/3 cup	1 starch/bread
Wheat germ	3 Tbsp.	1 starch/bread
Lean Meat		
Bacon substitute	2 Tbsp.	1 lean meat
Brewer's yeast	2 level Tbsp.	1 lean meat
Cheeses: See Chapter Five		
Dried beans and peas, cooked		
Black beans (turtle beans)	1 cup	2 starch/bread 1 lean meat

Food	Quantity	Exchanges
Black-eyed peas (cowpeas)	1 cup	2 starch/bread 1 lean meat
Broad beans (Faba beans)	2/3 cup	2 starch/bread 1 lean meat
Calico	1 cup	2 starch/bread 1 lean meat
Garbanzo, chickpeas	2/3 cup	2 starch/bread 1 lean meat
Kidney	1 cup	2 starch/bread 1 lean meat
Lentils	1 cup	2 starch/bread 1 lean meat
Lima	1 cup	2 starch/bread 1 lean meat
Mung	2 cups	1 starch/bread 1 lean meat
Navy	2/3 cup	2 starch/bread 1 lean meat
Pinto	2/3 cup	2 starch/bread 1 lean meat
Split peas	2/3 cup	2 starch/bread 1 lean meat
Split pea soup	1 cup	2 starch/bread 1 lean meat
Textured vegetable protein	3/4 oz.	1/2 starch/bread 1 lean meat

Medium Fat Meat

Cheeses: See Chapter Five

Soybeans	1/3 cup	1/2 starch/bread 1 med. fat meat
Tofu	1/2 cup (4 oz.)	1 med. fat meat

High Fat Meat Exchanges

Cheeses: See Chapter Five

Hommous	1 Tbsp.	1 starch/bread 1 high fat meat

Nuts

Almonds	1/4 cup (1 oz.)	1 high fat meat 1 fat
Brazil nuts	1/4 cup (1 oz.)	1 high fat meat 2 fat
Butternuts	1/4 cup (1 oz.)	1 high fat meat 1 fat

Food	Quantity	Exchanges
Peanuts, roasted	1/4 cup (6 oz.)	1 high fat meat 1 fat
Pecans	1/4 cup (1 oz.)	1 high fat meat 1 fat
Pignolias, Pinenut	2 Tbsp.	1 high fat meat 1 fat
Pistachio	60 nuts (1 oz.)	1 high fat meat 1 fat
Walnuts	16-20 halves (1 oz.)	1 high fat meat 1 fat
Peanut butter	1 Tbsp.	1 high fat meat
Seeds		
Pumpkin or squash seeds	1/4 cup	1 high fat meat 1 fat
Sesame seeds	1/4 cup	1 high fat meat 1 fat
Sunflower seeds	1/4 cup	1 high fat meat 1 fat
Sunflower seeds with hulls	1/2 cup	1 high fat meat 1 fat

For exchange values of meat analogs, consult the nutrient analysis provided by the companies selling the products. Commercial meat analogs are very high in sodium. Nutritional analyses are available from Loma Linda Foods, Riverside, California 92505, and Worthington Foods, Miles Lab, Worthington, Ohio 43085. A few choices are listed here.

Food	Quantity	Exchanges
Vegetable Protein Foods		
Big Franks	3/4 frank	1 lean meat
Breakfast strips	3 strips	2 fat
Breakfast links	3 links	1 high fat meat
Breakfast patties	1 patty	1 high fat meat
Chicken style slices	1½ slices	1 high fat meat
Chicken, fried	2 avg.	1/2 starch/bread 2 med. fat meat 2 fat
Chili (canned)	1/2 cup	1 starch/bread 1 med. fat meat 1 vegetable
Choplets	1 piece (1½ oz.)	1 lean meat

Food	Quantity	Exchanges
Dinner cuts	2 slices	2 lean meat
Griddle steaks	1/2 steak	1 high fat meat
Vege-Burger	1/2 cup	3 lean meat
Vegetarian Burgery (canned)	1/3 cup	1/2 starch/bread 2 lean meat
Vegetarian Nuteena	1 slice	1 med. fat meat 2 fat
Vegetarian Prosage	4 avg. (4 links)	2 med. fat meat 3 fat
Vegetarian Tender Bits	4 avg.	1 med. fat meat
Vegetarian Vegeloma	1 slice	2 lean meat
Vegetable		
Bamboo shoots, cooked	1 cup	1 vegetable
Bean sprouts		
Alfalfa	1 cup raw, 3/4 cup cooked	1 vegetable
Mung	1 cup raw, 3/4 cup cooked	1 vegetable
Soy	1 cup raw, 3/4 cup cooked	1 vegetable
Carrot juice	1/4 cup	1 vegetable
Water chestnuts, canned	6 whole	1 vegetable
Milk		
Goat's milk	1 cup	1 skim milk 2 fat
Kefir	1 cup	1 skim milk 2 fat
Soy milk, fortified	1 cup	1/2 med. fat meat 1/2 skim milk
Yogurt	1 cup	1 low fat milk
Fat		
Lecithin	2 tsp.	1 fat
Tahini sesame paste	1 tsp.	1 fat
Free		
Carob powder	1 Tbsp.	free
Sprouts, alfalfa, mung, or soy	1/2 cup	free

Word List

Brewer's yeast: A savory flavoring in powdered form used as a supplement in cooking. It does not rise like regular yeast.

Buckwheat: A bushlike plant. Buckwheat seeds are called groats; coarse ground groats are grits; and finely ground groats are buckwheat flour.

Hommous: A spread made from pureed garbanzo beans, tahini, lemon juice and spices.

Kasha: Cooked or roasted groats.

Kefir: A cultured dairy product similar to milk.

Legumes: Dried beans such as kidney, garbanzo, navy, pinto, lima, soybeans, peanuts, black-eyed peas, chick peas and lentils.

Meat analogs: Vegetable protein foods that duplicate the flavor, texture and appearance of meat.

Miso: Soybean paste.

Soymeat: Spun soy protein products. The cheese-like curd from soybeans is sent through many mechanical manipulations in order to obtain the texture of the final product.

Tahini: Sesame seed paste.

Tempeh: Soybean derivative; contains protein and carbohydrates.

Tofu: Soft unripened cheese-like curd made from soybeans.

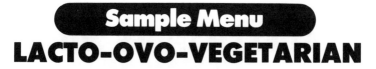

LACTO-OVO-VEGETARIAN

	Meal Plan (Exchanges)	Menu (Foods)
Breakfast:	3 Starch/Bread	2 slices whole wheat toast 1/2 cup cooked oats
	1 Fruit	1/2 cup orange juice
	1 Milk	1 cup skim milk
	2 Fat	2 tsp. margarine
Snack:	1 Fruit or Starch/Bread	1 apple or 6 whole wheat crackers
Lunch:	2 Starch/Bread	1 pita bread, 1/2 cup garbanzo spread
	2 Meat	(1 lean meat from garbanzo spread) 1/4 cup cottage cheese
	0 to 1 Vegetable	Diced tomatoes, shredded lettuce, diced onions
	1 Fruit	1 medium orange
	1 Milk	1 cup skim milk
	1 Fat	1 tsp. tahini paste
Snack:	1 Starch/Bread	4 squares Ry Krisp
	1 Fruit	1/2 banana
Dinner:	3 Starch/Bread 2 Meat 1 Vegetable	1/2 cup spaghetti (1 Starch/Bread) 1 cup lentil spaghetti sauce (2 Starch/Bread, 2 Lean Meat, 1 Vegetable)
	1 Vegetable	Green salad with bean sprouts
	1 Fruit	1 slice pineapple with juice
	1 Fat	1 Tbsp. French dressing
Snack:	1 Starch/Bread	3 cups popcorn
	1 Milk	1 cup skim milk
	0-1 Fat	1 tsp. margarine
Total:	2000 calories	275 grams carbohydrate (57%) 88 grams protein (18%) 55 grams fat (25%)

Chapter Fifteen
EAT EXCHANGES WITH CHOPSTICKS

Oriental cooking has become popular. If you enjoy cooking oriental dishes or frequent Chinese, Japanese or Korean restaurants, the following exchange lists should help you.

Chinese cooking involves much food preparation, but the actual cooking time is brief. Cooking methods are steaming, boiling or stir-frying in a small amount of hot fat. Milk and cheese are rarely used and meats are used in small quantities. A wide variety of vegetables is included. Fruits are considered a delicacy. A main meal usually consists of soup, hot rice, and several platters of vegetables and meats which can be shared by all who are at the table.

The Japanese also use a large variety of vegetables along with many kinds of fish. Main dishes are a combination of meat and vegetables seasoned with soy sauce. A variety of fresh fruit is eaten and white rice is the staple food item. Soy sauce is used to season and flavor food along with miso sauce, a soybean product.

Deep fat frying of fish, shellfish and vegetables (tempura) is one of the few times when fat is used in food preparation. Also popular are simple cakes and cookies, made of sugar and rice flour, that contain little or no fat. Usually desserts are not part of an oriental meal. However, sugar is often used in cooking Japanese dishes such as sukiyaki, teriyaki, and sushi.

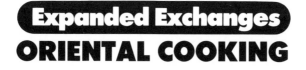

ORIENTAL COOKING

Food	Quantity	Exchanges
Starch/Bread		
Arrowroot starch	2 Tbsp.	1 starch/bread
Bow (Chinese steamed dough)	1 small or 2/3 medium	1 starch/bread
Cellophane noodles, cooked	1/2 cup	1 starch/bread
Chow mein noodles	1/2 cup	1 starch/bread 1 fat
Chestnuts	4 large, 6 small	1 starch/bread
Cornstarch	2 Tbsp.	1 starch/bread
Congee rice soup	1 cup	1 starch/bread
Egg roll wrapper	2	1 starch/bread
Fried rice	1/2 cup	1 starch/bread 2 fat
Ginkgo seeds	1½ oz.	1 starch/bread
Glutinous rice	1/3 cup	1 starch/bread
Glutinous rice flour	2 Tbsp.	1 starch/bread
Miso	3 Tbsp.	1 starch/bread
Mung bean noodles	1/2 cup	1 starch/bread
Mung bean starch sheets	1/2 cup	1 starch/bread
Poi	1/3 cup	1 starch/bread
Rice, cooked (loosely packed)	1/3 cup	1 starch/bread
Won ton wrappers, 3″ × 3″	4	1 starch/bread
Won ton, fried	3	1 starch/bread 4 fat
Wheat fritters	1 oz.	1 starch/bread
Meat		
Lean Meat Exchanges		
Abalone	1 oz.	1 lean meat
Chicken wings	1 wing	1 lean meat
Red mung beans	1/3 cup	1 starch/bread 1 lean meat

Food	Quantity	Exchanges
Horse beans, broad beans	1/3 cup	1 starch/bread 1 lean meat
Octopus	1¾ oz.	1 lean meat
Shrimp, dried	1/2 oz.	1 lean meat
Squid	1/2 cup (1¾ oz.)	1 lean meat
Medium Fat Meat Exchanges		
Dried curd sheet	1 oz.	1 med. fat meat
Duck feet	3	1 med. fat meat
Egg flower soup	2 cups	1 med. fat meat
Fish maw	2 oz.	1 med. fat meat
Oxtail	1 oz.	1 med. fat meat
Tofu curd ("dowfu")	4 oz.	1 med. fat meat
High Fat Meat Exchanges		
Anchovies	10	1 high fat meat
Chinese sausage	1 oz.	1 high fat meat
Eel	1 oz.	1 high fat meat
Pork feet	2 oz.	1 high fat meat 1 fat
Preserved duck egg	2/3 egg	1 high fat meat
Vegetable		
Arrowroot, 2" in diameter	1	1 vegetable
Bok choy	1 cup cooked	1 vegetable
Bamboo shoots, canned, diced	1 cup	1 vegetable
Bean sprouts	1 cup raw, 3/4 cup cooked	1 vegetable
Chayote (pear squash)	1/2 medium	1 vegetable
Chinese cabbage	2 cups raw, 1 cup cooked	1 vegetable
Chinese eggplant	1/2 cup	1 vegetable
Coriander (Chinese parsley)	1 cup	1 vegetable
Daikon (Chinese radish)	1 cup	1 vegetable
Ginger	1/4 cup	1 vegetable
Kohlrabi	2/3 cup	1 vegetable
Leek (Chinese onion)	1/2 cup or 2 medium	1 vegetable
Lotus root	1/2 cup	1 vegetable
Lotus seeds	1 oz.	1 vegetable

Food	Quantity	Exchanges
Bitter melon	1/2 cup	1 vegetable
Fuzzy melon	1/2 cup	1 vegetable
Miso	1 Tbsp.	1 vegetable
Button or straw mushrooms	1/2 cup	1 vegetable
Dried black mushrooms	1/4 cup	1 vegetable
Mustard leaves	1/2 cup	1 vegetable
Seaweed laver, soaked	1/2 cup	1 vegetable
Seahair, soaked	1/2 cup	1 vegetable
Snow peas	1/2 cup	1 vegetable
Taro root	1/4 cup	1 vegetable
Water chestnuts	6 whole	1 vegetable

Fruits

Food	Quantity	Exchanges
Dried salted apricots	6 halves	1 fruit
Almond cookie	2	1 starch/bread or 1 fruit
Fortune cookie	2	1 starch/bread or 1 fruit
Carambala (star fruit)	1½	1 fruit
Red dates	6	1 fruit
Guava, fresh	1/2 cup or 1	1 fruit
Kumquats, fresh	5	1 fruit
Longans, raw	31	1 fruit
Loquats	12	1 fruit
Lychees, fresh, canned or dried	1/2 cup (10)	1 fruit
Fresh persimmon	2	1 fruit

Fat

Food	Quantity	Exchanges
Chicken fat or pork fat	1 tsp.	1 fat
Coconut cream	2 Tbsp.	1 fat
Coconut, grated	2 Tbsp.	1 fat
Macadamia nuts	3	1 fat
Pork, cured (Chinese)	1" cube	1 fat
Sesame or peanut oil	1 tsp.	1 fat
Sesame seeds	1 Tbsp.	1 fat
Watermelon seeds	1/3 oz.	1 fat

Food	Quantity	Exchanges
Free		
Garlic		
Ginger		
Vinegar		
Green onion		
Curry		
Star anise		
Hot mustard		
Combination Dishes		
Beef, chicken, or pork chow mein	2 cups	2 starch/bread 2-3 med. fat meat 1 vegetable 1 fat
Beef and vegetables	1½ cups	2 starch/bread 3 med. fat meat 1 vegetable
Chop Suey	1½ cups	1 starch/bread 3 med. fat meat
Chow Luny Aas (lobster tails in garlic sauce)	3/4 cup	3 med. fat meat 1 fat
Dim Sum		
Har-Gow	3 pieces	1/2 starch/bread 1/2 med. fat meat
Siu-Mai	2 pieces	1/2 starch/bread 1 med. fat meat
Gow-Gee	3 pieces	1 starch/bread 1 med. fat meat
War-Tip	2 pieces	1/2 starch/bread 1 med. fat meat
Egg Drop Soup	1 cup	free
Egg Foo Young	1 medium patty	2 med. fat meat 1 vegetable 2 fat
Egg Foo Young Sauce	1/4 cup	1 vegetable
Egg Roll	1	1 starch/bread 1 med. fat meat 1 vegetable
Fried rice (rice, meat, eggs, onion)	1 cup	1 starch/bread 1 med. fat meat 1 vegetable 1 fat

Food	Quantity	Exchanges
Fung Gawn Aar (shrimp, chicken liver, mushrooms in chicken broth)	1 cup	3 med. fat meat 2 fat
Moo Goo Gai Pan	1½ cups	3 med. fat meat 1 vegetable 2 fat
Mum Yee Mein (braised noodles, breast of chicken, mushrooms, chestnuts, Chinese peas)	1 cup	2 starch/bread 2 med. fat meat 1 fat
Pepper steak	1 cup	1 starch/bread 3 med. fat meat 1 vegetable
Ramaki (chicken livers, water chestnuts, wrapped in bacon)	2 pieces	1 med. fat meat 1 fat
Shiu Mi (chopped chestnuts, chives, pork wrapped in thin noodles)	2 pieces	1/2 starch/bread 1/2 fat
Sukiyaki	1½ cups	3 med. fat meat 1 fat
Sweet and sour pork	1 cup	1 starch/bread 2 med. fat meat 1 vegetable 1 fruit 2 fat
with rice	1/2 cup	1 starch/bread
Won ton, boiled	4	1 starch/bread 1 med. fat meat 1 fat
Won ton soup	2 won tons and broth	1 starch/bread 1 fat

Word List

Bean curd, Tofu:	Smooth, creamy, custard-like product, made by pureeing soybeans.
Bean sprouts:	Tiny white shoots with pale green hoods.
Bitter melon:	Cucumber-like vegetable with a bitter flavor.
Congee:	A thin rice gruel.

Dim sum:	Steamed or fried dumplings stuffed with meat, seafood and/or vegetables, sweet paste or preserves.
Duck feet:	Duck feet braised in soy sauce, sugar, wine, salt, monosodium glutamate and spices.
Duck eggs:	Duck eggs soaked in brine for 30 to 40 days.
Egg roll:	Minced or shredded meat and/or seafood and vegetables wrapped in egg roll wrapper and deep fried.
Fish maw:	Dried and deep fried stomach lining of fish.
Ginkgo nuts:	Small fruit of Ginkgo tree with tough, beige colored shells and ivory colored nuts.
Kumquat:	Tiny oval shaped, yellow-orange citrus fruit.
Loquats:	Smooth, yellow-orange fruit.
Lotus root:	Tuberous stem of the water lily.
Lychee:	Also spelled lichee, or litchee, a small delicate, juicy, round fruit.
Noodles, cellophane:	Hard, opaque, fine white noodles made from ground mung beans.
Rice, glutinous:	Short grained, opaque, pearl white rice. It becomes sticky when cooked.
Taro:	Starchy, tuberous, rough textured brown root.
Won ton:	Wrapper filled with minced pork, shrimp and green onion.
Won ton wrapper:	Thin, yellow sheets made of flour, egg, salt and water.

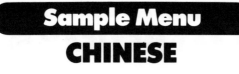

CHINESE

Menu (Foods)	Meal Plan (Exchanges)
Chicken Chow mein 2 cups	2 starch/bread 2 medium fat meat 1 vegetable 1 fat
Chow mein noodles 1/2 cup	1 starch/bread 1 fat
Steamed rice 1/3 cup	1 starch/bread
Fortune cookie two	1 fruit
Total:	4 starch/bread 2 medium fat meat 1 vegetable 1 fruit 2 fat

If your meal plan does not include all these exchanges you must make some decisions. See chapter 15 for guidelines.

Chapter Sixteen
OLE! EAT MEXICAN STYLE

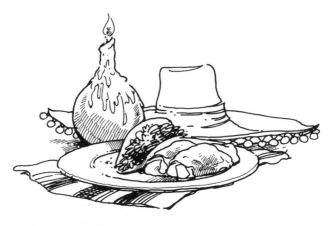

To add spice and variety to your eating, try some of the dishes from our neighbors south of the border. The southwestern part of the United States is a unique blending of several cultural backgrounds—Anglo, Indian, Mexican and Spanish. A melding of food habits has resulted in Mexican-American foods.

Beans are a staple food and are found in many dishes and combinations. Chicken, beef, eggs and potatoes are frequently used. Fresh tomatoes and chilis made from green and red peppers are also popular. Tortillas are a bread item often included in Mexican meals.

You need to be alert to the use of lard, salt pork and bacon fat in Mexican cooking. When preparing Mexican foods yourself, make appropriate substitutions for these saturated fats. Although Mexican foods are the main focus of this chapter you may also find some common Spanish foods also included.

Expanded Exchanges
MEXICAN COOKING

Food	Quantity	Exchanges
Starch/Bread		
Breadfruit	2 pieces, 2″ × 1″ wedge	1 starch/bread
Cassava	1/2 cup	1 starch/bread

Food	Quantity	Exchanges
Corn, taco or tortilla chips	1 cup (1 oz.)	1 starch/bread 2 fat
Dahl	1/2 cup	1 starch/bread
Hominy	1/2 cup	1 starch/bread
"Hops" bread	1 small	1 starch/bread
Jicama	1 cup (1/2 cup = 1 vegetable)	1 starch/bread
Malanga	1/2 cup	1 starch/bread
Masa harina	2 Tbsp.	1 starch/bread
Mexican style beans in a bowl (frijoles in a bowl)	1/2 cup	1 starch/bread 1 fat
Plantain, mature, cooked	1/3	1 starch/bread
Plantain, green, 11″ long	1/4	1 starch/bread
Refried beans (Frijoles refritos)	1/3 cup	1 starch/bread 2 fat
Hard roll, 3″	1	1 starch/bread
Hard roll, 6″	1/3	1 starch/bread
Spanish rice	1/3 cup	1 starch/bread 1 fat
Taco shell, 6″ diameter	2	1 starch/bread 1 fat
Thin tortillas		
Corn tortilla, 6″	1	1 starch/bread
Flour tortilla, 7″	1	1 starch/bread
Flour tortilla, 12″	1/2	1 starch/bread
Vermicelli	1/3 cup	1 starch/bread
Yam, white	1/3 cup	1 starch/bread
Yautia	1 small or 1/3 cup boiled	1 starch/bread
Meat		
Skirt steak	1 oz.	1 lean meat
Queso fresco	1 oz.	1 med. fat meat
Queso Mexican	1 oz.	1 med. fat meat
Queso "Jalisco"	1 oz.	1 med. fat meat
Goat	4 small cubes	1 med. fat meat
Mexican style sausage Chorizo, beef or pork	1 oz.	1 high fat meat
Vegetable		
Calabazita, Mexican squash	1/2 cup	1 vegetable

Food	Quantity	Exchanges
Chayote (squash)	1/2 cup	1 vegetable
Cactus leaves (nopales)	1/2 cup	1 vegetable
Hot chili pepper (Jalapeno)	4 peppers	1 vegetable
Ensalada de Aquacite, sliced avocado with tomato and lettuce	1/2 cup	1 vegetable 3 fat
Jicama	1/2 cup	1 vegetable
Gazpacho	1/2 cup	1 vegetable 1 fat
Okra	1/2 cup	1 vegetable
Tomatoes, small green	1/2 cup or 2	1 vegetable
Verdolages (Purslane)	1/2 cup	1 vegetable

Fruit

Food	Quantity	Exchanges
Cherimoya	1/2 small	1 fruit
Guava	1	1 fruit
Apple banana	1/2 medium	1 fruit
Cactus fruit	1 medium	1 fruit
Coco plum	1 medium	1 fruit
Mamey	1/2 medium	1 fruit
Mango	1/2	1 fruit
Guava nectar	1/2 cup	1 fruit
Papaya	1 cup	1 fruit
Sapote (custard apple)	1 small	1 fruit
Spanish sauce	1/2 cup	1 fruit 1 fat
Tamarind	12	1 fruit

Fat

Food	Quantity	Exchanges
Ackee (Jamaican)	3 pieces	1 fat
Avocado, 4" diameter	1/8	1 fat
Ghee	1 tsp.	1 fat
Guacamole	2 Tbsp.	1 fat
Sofrito	2 tsp.	1 fat

Free Foods

Amaranthus
Chile salsa
Fresh cilantro

Food	Quantity	Exchanges
Combination Dishes		
Beef cubes in brown gravy (Carne Guisada)	1 cup	1/2 starch/bread 2 lean meat 2 fat
Burrito de carne (meat with flour tortilla) (If deep fat fried add extra fat)	1 small, 7" tortilla	1½ starch/bread 2 med. fat meat 1 fat
	1 large, 9" tortilla	3 starch/bread 3 med. fat meat 1 fat
Burrito de frijoles refritos (beans with flour tortilla) (If deep fat fried add extra fat)	1 small, 7"	3 starch/bread 1 med. fat meat 1 fat
	1 large, 9"	4 starch/bread 1½ med. fat meat 2 fat
Chili con carne without beans	1 cup	1/2 starch/bread 3 med. fat meat
Chili con carne with beans	1 cup	1½ starch/bread 3 med. fat meat 1 fat
Chili rellenos	7"	2 starch/bread 2 med. fat meat 1 vegetable 2 fat
Chili verde (diced meat, green chili, rice or beans)	1 cup	1 starch/bread 3 med. fat meat 1 vegetable 2 fat
Corn fritters	1 serving	1 starch/bread 2 med. fat meat 1 fat
Enchiladas, beef (6" tortilla, ground beef, mozzarella cheese, red chili sauce)	1	1½ starch/bread 2 med. fat meat 1 fat
Enchiladas, cheese (6" tortilla, mozzarella cheese, red chili sauce)	1	1½ starch/bread 1 to 2 med. fat meat 2 fat
Flauta (rolled, filled fried corn tortilla)	1	1 starch/bread 1 med. fat meat

Food	Quantity	Exchanges
Mexican or Spanish rice (rice, tomato sauce, green chilis)	1/2 cup	1 starch/bread 1 vegetable 1 fat
Picadillo	3/4 cup	1 starch/bread 2 med. fat meat 2 fat
Quesadillas (6" corn or 7" flour tortilla, green chilis, mozzarella cheese)	1	1 starch/bread 2 med. fat meat 2 fat
Rice with chicken (arroz con pollo)	3/4 cup	1 starch/bread 2 med. fat meat 1 fat
Mexican squash with beef (calabazita con carne)	1/2 cup	1 med. fat meat 1 vegetable 1 fat
Yellow squash and chicken	3/4 cup	2 lean meat 1 vegetable 2 fat
Open taco (tortilla, ground beef, lettuce, chili sauce)	1	1 starch/bread 3 med. fat meat 1 vegetable
Taco (7" tortilla, meat, cheese, tomato, lettuce)	1	1 starch/bread 1 or 2 med. fat meat 1 fat
Beef tamales with sauce	2 small or 1 large	2 starch/bread 1 to 2 med. fat meat 2 fat
Tostada or tortilla with refried beans	1 small	2 starch/bread 1 fat
Tostada with meat	1 small	1 starch/bread 1 med. fat meat 1 fat
Tostada, beef	1 large	2 starch/bread 2 med. fat meat 2 fat
Vermicelli or rice with beef (Fidelio con carne)	1 cup	2 starch/bread 2 med. fat meat 1 fat

Arroz con pollo:	Browned rice with chicken, tomatoes and spices.
Burrito:	A soft flour tortilla filled with beans or ground beef. It is rolled and covered with an enchilada sauce or deep fried.
Calabazita: (Mexican squash)	Similar in size and shape to the cucumber, except the skin is a light green. Simmered with onion and spices and often combined with meat in a casserole dish.
Calabazita con pollo:	Mexican squash with chicken.
Calabazita con carne:	Mexican squash with beef.
Carne guisada: (Beef tips in brown gravy)	Beef tips sauteed with chopped onions, green pepper and chili peppers. Stewed tomatoes are added and the combination is simmered until tender.
Cassava: (Yucca root)	Starchy root, also called "manioc." It has a bitter odor that disappears after cooking. It is not eaten raw.
Chili:	Any variety of hot peppers, used raw or as an ingredient in sauces or dishes.
Chili relleno:	Juicy green chili pepper filled with cheese and wrapped in a rich egg batter. Deep fried and smothered in chili verde.
Chili verde:	Mixture of diced meat, green chili, rice or beans.
Chorizo:	A highly seasoned sausage of chopped beef or pork with sweet red peppers. The preparation is fried and eaten in a taco, burrito or tortilla mixed with scrambled eggs.
Cilantro:	The fresh leaves and stems of coriander, it imparts a distinctive flavor to salsa, meat dishes and soups.
Enchilada:	Oil blanched corn tortilla folded (or rolled) around a filling of beef or cheese. It can be covered with a sauce of chili con carne,

	tomato, cheese or guacamole and garnished with chopped onions or grated cheese.
Fidelio con carne:	Sauteed beef cubes combined with browned vermicelli, tomatoes and spices.
Frijoles in a bowl: (Mexican style beans in a bowl)	Beans are served in some form at every meal in Mexico. They are simmered until tender with onion, cilantro, chili pepper, diced tomatoes and seasonings.
Frijoles refritos:	Popularly known as refried beans. Beans are simmered with bacon, onion, garlic, whole tomatoes, cilantro and herbs until soft. Then they are mashed and fried slowly. Chili powder may be added.

Fruit:

Cherimoya:	It has a rough green outer skin. When ripened and chilled, the flesh has a sherbet-like texture.
Guava:	A sweet juicy fruit ranging in color from green to yellow with red or yellow flesh.
Plantain:	Greenish looking banana with rough skin and a number of blemishes. It is used as a vegetable rather than a fruit because the fruit remains starchy, even when fully ripe. Never eaten raw.
Sapote:	Also called the Mexican custard apple. Clusters of the fruit are large, greenish-yellow. They resemble green apples in appearance.
Tamarind:	The fruit is a long, flattened pod, cinnamon brown in color.
Guacamole:	Avocado dip made with chopped chili and other seasonings.
Jicama:	The outside skin is tan; the inside, white. It is crisp and juicy with a water chestnut flavor. As familiar to Mexico as the potato is to the U.S.
Malanga:	Large herb with starchy, thick, tuberous, white edible root.
Nopales: (Cactus)	The leaves or pods of the prickly pear cactus are used. They taste like crisp green beans.

	They are sliced in strips and cooked with onions and spices.
Quesadillas:	Tortillas filled with cheese and heated or fried until cheese melts. They are eaten with salsa, usually as snacks.
Queso fesco:	White, crumbly Mexican cheese which is low in fat.
Salsa:	Chili sauce, served as an accompaniment.
Spanish rice:	White rice sauteed in a skillet with tomatoes, green peppers, onions and seasonings.
Taco:	A crisp, deep fat fried corn tortilla folded in half to hold seasoned ground beef, diced tomatoes, shredded lettuce and cheese.
Tortilla:	Baked, flat, round thin cakes of unleavened cornmeal (masa) or flour. The bread of Mexico.
Tamales, beef:	**Extruded cooked corn masa wrapped around a chili beef filling. A sauce of chili** con carne, tomato or cheese can be used as an accompaniment.
Tostadas:	Tortillas that have been fried until golden brown and crisp in hot lard or oil. They are then cooked with various combinations of meat, poultry, sauces, chilis, lettuce and tomatoes.

With a Mexican menu, chances are good you will need to make decisions: Choose what to eat, what to take home in a "doggie bag" or what to leave if everything does not fit into your meal plan.

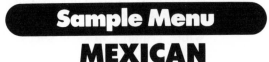

Sample Menu
MEXICAN

Menu (Foods)	Meal Plan (Exchanges)
Cheese Enchilada 1	1½ starch/bread 2 medium fat meat 2 fat
Beef Taco 1	1 starch/bread 2 medium fat meat 1 fat
Bean Tostada 1	2 starch/bread
Refried Beans 1/3 cup	1 starch/bread 1 fat
Spanish Rice 1/3 cup	1 starch/bread 1 fat
Total:	6½ starch/bread 4 medium fat meat 5 fat

Chapter Seventeen
MAMA MIA!
EXCHANGES ITALIANO

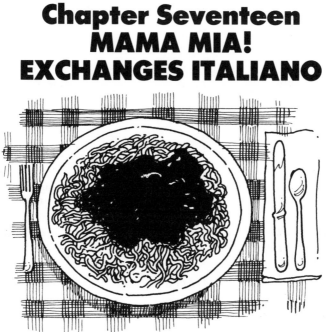

Italian cuisine has become another regular part of the American diet. Let's look at how it can be incorporated into the exchange meal plan.

Pasta is the staple of the Italian diet and is considered the "starchy" part of the meal. Italian bread is also eaten at every meal. Large quantities of vegetables, both cooked and raw, are used frequently; peppers and tomatoes are especially popular. Eggplant and zucchini are other favorite vegetables. Cheese is frequently used along with highly seasoned meats, such as sausages and salami. All types of fish are also used. Olive oil is the preferred cooking oil, and Italian foods are usually highly seasoned.

Expanded Exchanges
ITALIAN COOKING

Food	Quantity	Exchanges
Starch/Bread		
Italian bread	1 slice (1 oz.)	1 starch/bread
Italian bread with garlic butter	1 slice (1 oz.)	1 starch/bread 1 fat

Food	Quantity	Exchanges
Minestrone soup	1 cup	1 starch/bread 1 fat
Pastas	1/2 cup	1 starch/bread
Vermicelli soup	1 cup	1 starch/bread
Meat		
Prosciutto (Italian ham)	1 oz.	1 med. fat meat
Provolone cheese	1 oz.	1 high fat meat
Meat balls	1 oz.	1 med. fat meat
Basic Italian cheese sauce (alfredo)	1/2 cup	1 high fat meat 1/2 milk 2 fat
Basic Italian tomato sauce with meat	1/2 cup	1 starch/bread 1 high fat meat
Vegetable		
Gazpacho	1/2 cup	1 vegetable 1 fat
Italian green beans (Romano)	1/2 cup	1 vegetable 1½ fat
Ratatouille	1/2 cup	1 vegetable 1 fat
Tomato paste	1 Tbsp.	1 vegetable
Tomato puree	1/4 cup	1 vegetable
Tomato sauce	1/3 cup	1 vegetable
Basic Italian tomato sauce, meatless	1/2 cup	1 vegetable 1 fat
Combination Dishes		
Cannelloni	4 stuffed noodles	2 starch/bread 4 med. fat meat 2 vegetable 2 fat
Chicken cacciatore	1/2 small chicken breast with sauce	3 lean meat 1 vegetable 1 fat
Chicken tetrazzini (Pollo alla tetrazzini)	1 cup	1½ starch/bread 2 med. fat meat
Eggplant parmigiana	1 cup	1 bread/starch 2 med. fat meat 2 vegetable 2 fat

Food	Quantity	Exchanges
Italian spaghetti with meat sauce	1 cup	2 starch/bread 1 med. fat meat 2 vegetable 1 fat
Italian spaghetti with meatballs (spaghetti con polpette)	1 cup (with 6 small meatballs)	2 starch/bread 2 med. fat meat 2 vegetable
Italian spaghetti with tomato sauce	1 cup	3 starch/bread 1 vegetable
Lasagna	1 serving (3" × 4")	1 starch/bread 3 med. fat meat 1 vegetable 1 fat
Manicotti	2 shells	3 starch/bread 3 med. fat meat 2 vegetable 2 fat
Pizza with cheese, sausage, pepperoni	1/4 of a 16 to 18 oz. pizza	2 starch/bread 2 med. fat meat 1 vegetable 1 fat
Ravioli with beef	1 cup	2 starch/bread 1 med. fat meat 1 vegetable
Ravioli with cheese	1 cup	2 starch/bread 1 med. fat meat 1 vegetable 1 fat
Veal parmigiana	1 cutlet	1 starch/bread 4 med. fat meat 1 vegetable 1 fat

Word List

Cannelloni:	Hollow pasta that is filled and served with cheese and tomato sauce.
Chicken cacciatore:	Sauteed chicken pieces simmered in a meatless tomato sauce.
Italian green beans: (Romano)	Wide, quick cooking green beans that are often served in a sauce.

Lasagna:	Very wide, flat pasta served with meat, cheese and tomato sauce.
Pasta:	Includes fettuccine, linguine, spaghetti, cannelloni, macaroni, elbow, shells, noodles, rigatoni, rotelle, vermicelli, etc.
Ravioli:	A pasta square stuffed with eggs, vegetables, cheese or meat and covered with tomato sauce.
Manicotti:	Large tubular pasta served with a filling of meat or cheese and with meatless tomato suace.
Veal parmigiana:	Thin slices of veal, pounded for tenderness, rolled in bread crumbs and Parmesan cheese, covered with mozzarella cheese and a meatless tomato sauce.

Sample Menu

ITALIAN

Menu (Foods)	Meal Plan (Exchanges)
Spaghetti with Mushrooms and Meat Balls 2 cups	4 starch/bread 4 medium fat meat 2 vegetable
Vegetable Tossed Salad with Italian Dressing	1 vegetable 2 fat
Italian Bread with Butter	1 starch/bread 1 fat
Total:	5 starch/bread 4 medium fat meat 3 vegetable 3 fat

Chapter Eighteen
JEWISH COOKERY

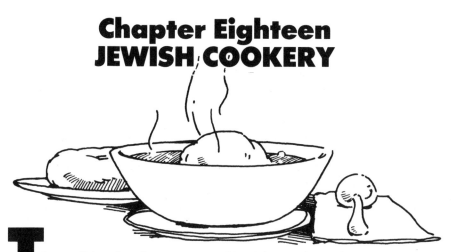

The traditional eating patterns of Jewish people are based on the Laws of Kashruth, which are the general dietary laws from the Torah, and on customs for the celebration of holidays. Kosher means "proper, fit" and refers to foods that can be eaten in accordance with Jewish dietary laws, including specific categories of foods and their selection. It also refers to the slaughter, preparation and service of meat, the separation of meat and dairy products, and the separation of cooking, serving, and eating utensils. These laws are observed in varying degrees by Orthodox, Conservative and Reformed denominations.

The word "traif", which describes animals found non-kosher because of physical damage or imperfections, is commonly used to describe all foods that are non-kosher.

A very important aspect of planning meals according to the laws of Kashruth is the prohibition against mixing meat (fleischig) or poultry with dairy foods (milchig).

Meats that come from animals that chew their curd, have split hooves and have been slaughtered in the manner prescribed by the Torah are acceptable. Cattle, sheep, goats, and deer fall into this category, but pork, pork products, and rabbit are not kosher. Chicken, duck, geese, and turkey are also acceptable.

Dairy and meat or poultry products may not be eaten at the same meal. A meal must contain either meat or dairy products. After eating meat, it is customary to wait six hours before eating dairy products. After eating a dairy meal, meat foods may be eaten after rinsing the mouth and a brief wait—often one-half to one hour.

Fish are considered "pareve" (neutral). Fish and meat may be eaten during the same meal but not together. Fish must have both fins and permanent scales to be kosher.

Fruits, vegetables, and eggs are also pareve. Pareve foods contain neither meat nor milk and are prepared in utensils used for pareve only. They can be served for either a milk or a meat meal.

Many breads, cakes, and cereals are kosher. They are a neutral food if milk, butter, or other dairy products or derivatives are not used.

Water rolls (bagels), rye and pumpernickel breads, and whole grains such as oatmeal, barley, brown rice and buckwheat groats (kasha) are used frequently. Soups, especially chicken noodle and chicken rice, are often used. Spinach or sorrel leaves are used for schav, a popular soup. Broccoli, carrots, sweet potatoes and yams, stuffed green peppers, fresh and canned tomatoes, cabbage and potatoes are used extensively. Cooked or dried fruits are commonly served and fresh or stewed fruits are often eaten as desserts with the meat meal.

Historically, the kosher diet has been high in fat. Many cuts of kosher meat are well-marbled with fat. Schmaltz (chicken fat) has been a favorite ingredient for many traditional Jewish dishes. It has been used for flavor and even as an ingredient for sandwiches. Margarine or kosher certified vegetable oil, which are pareve (neutral, containing no milk or meat ingredients) can be substituted in smaller amounts.

Fried dishes also have been popular in kosher cooking. Blintzes (crepes) and matzo brie (fried matzo) are examples. However, in place of using schmaltz or butter, small amounts of vegetable oil can be used.

Many traditional dishes are also high in sodium. The koshering process is a salting process, and kosher meats and poultry tend to be high in sodium. Fresh kosher fish does not have to be salted to be kosher.

In preparing you own dishes, substitutes for high saturated fat and high salt products can be used.

Expanded Exchanges
JEWISH COOKING

Food	Quantity	Exchanges
Bread		
Bagel	1/2	1 starch/bread
Bialy (Roll)	1/2 (1 oz.)	1 starch/bread
Buckwheat groats (kasha), cooked	1/3 cup	1 starch/bread

Food	Quantity	Exchanges
Bulke (roll)	1/2	1 starch/bread
Challah	1 slice or 1 oz.	1 starch/bread
Farfel	3 Tbsp.	1 starch/bread
Hard roll (kaiser)	1/2	1 starch/bread
Kichel, 1" square	3	1 starch/bread
Lukshen (noodles, etc.)	1/2 cup, cooked	1 starch/bread
Matzo, 6' diameter	1	1 starch/bread
Matzo crackers, 1½" square	7	1 starch/bread
Matzo meal	2½ Tbsp.	1 starch/bread
Matzo balls (knadlach)	1	1 starch/bread 1 fat
Matzo meal pancakes	1	1 starch/bread 2 fat
Matzo kugel	1/2 serving	1 starch/bread 1 fat
Potato kugel	1/2 cup	1 starch/bread 1 fat
Potato knish, 3" round	2	1 starch/bread 2 fat
Potato latkes	1/2 cup raw batter	1 starch/bread 1 fat
Potato starch	2 Tbsp.	1 starch/bread
Meat		
Beef tongue	1 oz.	1 med. fat meat
Caviar	1 oz.	1 lean meat
Chopped liver	1 oz.	1 high fat meat
Corned beef	1 oz.	1 high fat meat
Flanken	1 oz.	1 high fat meat 1 fat
Gefilte fish	1 oz.	1 lean meat
Kippered herring	1 oz.	1 lean meat
Lox (smoked salmon)	1 oz.	1 lean meat
Pot cheese	1/4 cup	1 lean meat
Pickled herring	1 oz.	1 lean meat
Sablefish	2 oz.	1 high fat meat
Stewed chicken	1 oz.	1 high fat meat
Vegetable		
Borscht (beet soup with sour cream)	1/2 cup	1 vegetable 1 fat

Food	Quantity	Exchanges
Sauerkraut	1/2 cup	1 vegetable
Sorrel (schav)	1/2 cup	1 vegetable
Fat		
Chicken fat (schmaltz)	1 tsp.	1 fat
Grebnes (schmaltz cracklings)	1 tsp.	1 fat
Combination Foods		
Cabbage-beet borscht	1 cup	1 starch/bread 1 fat
Cheese Blintzes	1	2 starch/bread 1 med. fat meat 1 fat
Chopped liver	2 oz.	2 med. fat meat
Cholent (with meat)	1 cup	2 starch/bread 2 med. fat meat 1 vegetable 2 fat
Meat Kreplach	2 small	1 starch/bread 2 med. fat meat
Stuffed Cabbage in Tomato Sauce	1 large roll	1 starch/bread 2 med. fat meat 1 vegetable
Sweet Potato Tzimmes	1/2 cup	1 starch/bread 1 fruit
Tzimmes with Carrots and Apples	1/2 cup	2 vegetable 1 fat

These traditional treats should be avoided. They are high in sugar and fat.

bubke (coffeecake)
hamantaschen (purim tart)
kuchen and mandel bread (cake)
lekach (honeycakes)
rugalah (strudel)
teiglach (pastry)

Bagel:	A hard yeast roll shaped like a doughnut.
Blintzes:	Very thin rolled pancakes usually filled with cottage or pot cheese or fruit mixture.
Borscht:	Beet soup served hot or cold.L
Bubke:	Coffee cake, usually sour cream.
Bulke:	Large, light yeast roll, softer than a bagel.
Challah:	a loaf of very light egg bread, most commonly braided and prepared especially for the Sabbath and holidays.
Cholent:	A slow-cooking stew; can be prepared with or without meat. Appropriate for a dairy meal.
Farfel:	Noodle dough grated into barley-sized grains and served in soup during Passover. Crumbled matzoh.
Fleisch:	A term describing meat and meat products.
Gefilte fish:	A highly seasoned chopped white fish mixture usually stuffed into the fish skin.
Hamantaschen:	Three-grained cakes with pastry or cookie crust and filled with poppy seeds, dried fruit, or cheese.
Kasha:	Buckwheat groats served as a cooked cereal or as a potato substitute with meat gravy.
Kashruth:	A noun describing the Kosher dietary laws based on the Torah.
Kichlach:	Light egg cookies.
Knaidlach or Kloese:	Dumplings in chicken soup.
Knishes:	Pastry filled with meat and spices. The pastry can have a potato base.
Kosher:	"Clean, proper, and fit to consume" foods. Describes foods and practices sanctioned by Jewish law.
Kreplach:	Bite-sized meat-filled pastry.
Kuchen:	Coffee cake.

Kugel:	Pudding. Common types are made with potatoes or noodles.
Latkes:	Pancakes, potatoes latkes are very popular.
Leckach:	Honey cake.
Lox:	Smoked and salted salmon that is cut very thin.
Lukshen:	Noodles.
Matzo:	Flat, unleavened cracker.
Matzoh Meal:	Finely ground matzoh used in cooking and baking.
Milchig:	A term describing milk or dairy foods from a kosher dairy.
Pareve:	A term describing neutral foods; neither meat nor dairy.
Pirogen (Piroshkes):	Pastry filled with meat, cheese, or meat stuffing.
Pot Cheese:	Cream cheese or other farmer-style cheese.
Schmaltz:	Chicken fat, often used in cooking or pastry making.
Strudel:	Thin pastry rolled up with fruit and nut filling.
Sorrel:	A member of the buckwheat family. Cooked as a green leafy vegetable.
Teiglach:	Small balls of sweet dough cooked in honey.
Traif:	Foods not allowed.
Tzimmes:	Rice pudding eaten as a main course. May be made with dried fruit, carrots and fat meat.

Sample Menu
JEWISH

Menu (Foods)	**Meal Plan** (Exchanges)
Challah, margarine, 1 slice	1 starch/bread 1 fat
Gefilte fish, 1 oz.	1 lean meat
Beet borscht, 1/2 cup	1 vegetable
Stewed chicken, 3 oz.	3 med. fat meat
Potato kugel, 1 cup	2 starch/bread 2 fat
Fruit compote, 1/2 cup	1 fruit
Total:	3 starch/bread 4 meat 1 vegetable 1 fruit 3 fat

Chapter Nineteen
LET'S GO CAMPING

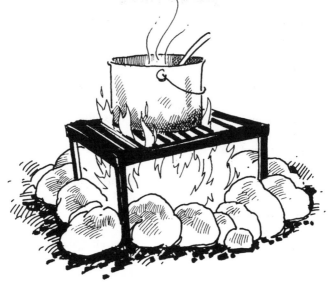

Camping is becoming more popular every year because it provides an opportunity to enjoy nature at its very best. Anyone who wants to experience this kind of life should jump into it with enthusiasm. Diabetes need not hold you back if you know how to prepare appropriately.

The preparation required will depend on the type of camping you plan to do. When camping with a motor home or camper trailer, nearly any type of food can be taken. Because campers are equipped with refrigeration and adequate storage areas for food and cooking utensils, food for this type of camping would be similar to that eaten at home.

Canoeing requires more special planning. Food must be compact, light-weight and nonperishable because it will need to be carried on portages and packed into confined areas of the canoe. Food should be filling and provide a concentrated source of nutrition.

Backpacking entails similar considerations. Everything, including a sleeping bag, cooking equipment and food, must be carried on your back. As with canoeing, space and weight are prime considerations, but food must also be filling and provide a concentrated source of nutrition.

For any type of camping, be sure to pack enough food for the duration of the trip. Experienced campers solve this problem by planning daily menus. Food for each meal can then be packed separately and labeled with the date and time it is to be eaten. The calculated amount should be increased slightly to ensure that enough food is taken in case a pack is lost or damaged. A camper with diabetes should never assume that fish or berries will be an available food source! You also need to be sure to take all your insulin and blood testing supplies and to wear medical identification.

Canoers, hikers or backpackers will need to increase their usual meal plan to allow for the increased activity. In general, begin by increasing calories by 20 percent; insulin requirements may be reduced as well. Check with your health care team about how much—it is generally a percentage of your total insulin dose often beginning with a 10 to 20 percent reduction in your total insulin dosage, reducing the insulin acting during the time of your activity. See the chapter on exercise for additional guidelines. Meal plans may need to be increased by as much as 1000 calories a day for very strenuous activity such as mountain backpacking. Snacks are always important, but even more so with this increased activity. Be sure to plan accordingly.

During hard hiking, lunch should be an all-day meal consumed in small, frequent installments to provide a steady flow of fuel without overloading the stomach. Weariness tends to kill the appetite, leading to a vicious cycle of deeper weariness and less appetite!

Freeze-dried and dried (dehydrated) foods can be used. Freeze-dried foods are the best because their flavor is more nearly like fresh foods and they are virtually foolproof in preparation—just add water and serve. When packaged in laminated aluminum foil and vacuum-sealed in plastic, they will last indefinitely. However, freeze-dried items are expensive. Dried foods should be discarded after one year.

Companies that manufacture freeze-dried products, such as Mountain House, Wilson & Company, Trail Chef, Oregon Freeze Dry Foods, Inc. and Rich-Moor Dehydrated Foods, will supply nutrition analysis of their products.

If milk is not available, or if you do not care for dried skim milk powder, substitute an extra meat, starch or fruit exchange for your milk exchange.

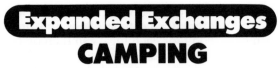
CAMPING

Food	Quantity	Exchanges
Starches		
Biscuits, 2″ square	1	1 starch/bread 1 fat
Chow mein noodles	1/2 cup	1 starch/bread 1 fat
Cooked cereal	1/2 cup	1 starch/bread
Corn	1/2 cup rehydrated or 1 oz. dried	1 starch/bread
Cornbread, 2″ square	1	1 starch/bread 1 fat
French toast	1	1 starch/bread 1/2 meat
Granola (See recipe in chapter 28)	1/4 cup	1 starch/bread 1 fat
Gorp (See recipe in chapter 28)	1/3 cup	1 starch/bread 1 fat
Granola bar	1 small bar	1 starch/bread 1 fat
Graham crackers	3 squares	1 starch/bread
Hash browns	1/2 cup or 2 oz. dried	1 starch/bread 1 fat
Hushpuppies, 2″ square	1	1 starch/bread 1 fat
Pancakes, 5″ diameter	1	1 starch/bread 1 fat
Pancakes, 4″ diameter	3	2 starch/bread 1 fat
Potatoes, mashed	1/2 cup or 3 oz. dried	1 starch/bread
Potatoes, diced	1/2 cup or 2 oz. dried	1 starch/bread
Rice	1/3 cup	1 starch/bread
Ry Krisp	3 triple crackers	1 starch/bread
Saltine crackers	6	1 starch/bread
Soups	1 cup	1 starch/bread
Vanilla wafers	6	1 starch/bread

Food	Quantity	Exchanges
Meat		
Beef jerky	1/2 oz.	1 lean meat
Beef	2 oz. dry weight	3 med. fat meat
Chicken	2 oz. dry weight	3 lean meat
Canned meat, (2 lb. can)	1/8 can	3 med. fat meat
Canned chicken (5 oz. can)	1/2 can	3 lean meat
Canned shrimp, sardines, etc.	1 oz.	1 lean meat
Cheese	1 oz.	1 high fat meat
Dried chipped beef (5 oz. can)	1/2 can	3 lean meat
Eggs, prepared	1/3 cup	2 med. fat meat
Eggs, dried	2 Tbsp.	1 med. fat meat
Ham	3 oz.	3 lean meat
Luncheon meat	1 slice (1 oz.)	1 high fat meat
Peanuts	1/4 cup (1 oz.)	**1 high fat meat 1 fat**
Peanut butter (comes in a tube)	1 Tbsp.	1 high fat meat
Pork chops	2 oz. dry weight	3 med. fat meat
Salami	1 oz. (1 slice, 1/4" thick)	1 high fat meat
Sausage patties	2 oz.	2 high fat meat
Spam	1 slice (3 oz.)	3 high fat meat
Sunflower seeds	1/4 cup (1 oz.)	1 high fat meat **1 fat**
Tuna fish, 7 oz. can	1/2 can	3 lean meat
Meat sticks	1/2 oz.	1 lean meat
Vegetable		
Carrots, green beans, spinach, etc.	1 oz. dried weight = 1/2 cup cooked	1 vegetable
Fruit		
Dried fruit	1/2 oz. (1/4 cup)	1 fruit
Fruit rolls or roll-ups	1 roll	**1 fruit**
Fruit bars	1 bar	1½ fruit
Fruit galaxie	1/4 cup	1 fruit
Fruit jerkey	1 strip	1 fruit
Juice	1/2 cup	1 fruit

Food	Quantity	Exchanges
Marshmallows, large	2	1 fruit
Prunes	3	1 fruit
Raisins	2 Tbsp. (1/2 oz.)	1 fruit
Stewed fruit	1/2 cup	1 fruit
Tang or other fruit drinks	1/2 cup prepared	1 fruit
Real maple syrup	1/4 cup	4 fruit
	1 Tbsp.	1 fruit
Maple syrup made with artificial sweeteners	1/4 cup	free

Milk

Dried nonfat milk powder	1/3 cup powder and 3/4 cup water	1 skim milk
Cocoa (See recipe in chapter 28)	1 cup	1 skim milk

Combination Foods

Baked beans and franks	1 cup	3 starch/bread 1 meat 1 fat
Beef stew	1 cup	2 starch/bread 2 meat 1 to 2 fat
Beef stroganoff	1 cup	2 starch/bread 2 meat 1 to 2 fat
Chicken a la king	1 cup	2 starch/bread 2 meat 1 to 2 fat
Chicken, beef or pork chow mein (without noodles or rice)	2 cups	1 starch/bread 2 meat 2 vegetable
Chicken with dumplings	1½ cups	1 starch/bread 1 vegetable 2 meat 1 fat
dumpling	1	1 starch/bread
Chili	1 cup	2 starch/bread 2 meat 1 fat
Lasagna	1 cup	1 starch/bread 3 meat 1 to 2 fat

Food	Quantity	Exchanges
Macaroni and cheese	1 cup	2 starch/bread 1 meat 2 fat
Spaghetti and meatballs	1 cup	2 starch/bread 2 meat 1 to 2 fat
Tuna noodle casserole with peas	1½ cups	2 starch/bread 1 vegetable 2 meat 1 fat

Desserts
(for occasional use)

Food	Quantity	Exchanges
Brownie, 2″ × 4″	1	2 starch/bread 2 fat
Cookies, 3″ diameter	1	1 starch/bread 1 fat
Cake, white or yellow, plain, no icing	3″ square	2 starch/bread 2 fat
Gingerbread	3″ × 2″	2 starch/bread
Pudding	1/2 cup	2 starch/bread

Fat

Food	Quantity	Exchanges
Margarine (comes in a tube)	1 tsp.	1 fat

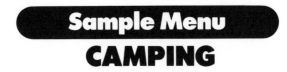
CAMPING

An example of a typical day's menu would allow for the following types of exchanges at each meal and snack time.

	Menu (Foods)	**Meal Plan** (Exchanges)
Breakfast:	Cooked cereals, biscuits, pancakes, French toast	Starch/Bread
	Dried egg powder	Meat
	Fruit juices or dried fruit	Fruit
	Cocoa	Milk
A.M. Snack:	Granola	Starch/Bread
Lunch:	Ry Krisp	Starch/Bread
	Hard salami, cheese, peanut butter	Meat
	Raisins	Fruit
	Artificially sweetened Kool-Aid	Free
Afternoon Snack:	Graham crackers, Ry Krisp, Gorp, granola bar	Starch/Bread
	Fruit Jerkey, raisins, dried fruit	Fruit
	Artificially sweetened Kool-Aid	Free
Dinner:	Biscuits or dessert	Starch/Bread
	Casseroles using starch/bread and meat exchanges	Meat
	Dried vegetables	Vegetable
	Dried fruit	Fruit
Evening Snack:	Crackers, biscuits, popcorn	Starch/Bread
	Cheese, peanuts, sunflower seeds	Meat
	Dried fruit	Fruit
	Dried milk or cocoa	Milk

Part III

GUIDELINES FOR
SPECIAL OCCASIONS

Chapter Twenty
UNDERSTAND YOUR MEAL PLAN AND ENJOY DINING OUT

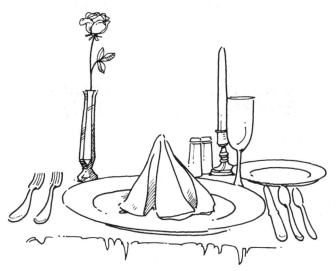

It has recently been reported that when Americans dine out—and they are doing this more than ever before—they aren't leaving their taste for a healthy diet at home. So if you have diabetes you have a lot of company from your friends and neighbors in making healthy food choices. In survey of consumers and restaurant managers conducted in 1986 by the National Restaurant Association, results showed patrons are eating more vegetables, less fat, less meat, and fewer fried foods than three years before. Consumers also continue to use less sugar and salt, more fish, and more salads. The Restaurant Association also estimates that more than 45 billion meals are eaten in restaurants, schools, and work cafeterias annually. On the average, each person eats out about 192 times a year.

In catering to customers' healthful preferences, the survey found, virtually all restaurants offer at least diet beverages (95%) or sugar substitutes (92%). Most also offer decaffeinated coffee, margarine, whole-grain bread, rolls, or crackers, and fresh fruit for dessert. About one-third offer reduced-calorie salad dressings, low fat or skim milk, salt substitutes, and bran cereals.

A growing number of restaurants are actively promoting nutrition or low-calorie fare. Almost three out of four restaurants will alter the way they prepare foods at a diner's request, the survey found. At least nine out of ten will serve a sauce or salad dressing on the side or cook without salt. Most also will cook with margarine or vegetable oil and help diners trying to limit saturated fats. Four out of five restaurants will broil or bake a food instead of frying it. It appears persons with diabetes have more help and choices available to them today.

When eating at a restaurant, cafeteria or a friend's home, bring your common sense with you. You can follow your meal plan and enjoy yourself at the same time. Knowledge of food values should enable anyone to select proper items in restaurants with fairly varied menus. For gastronomical adventures, follow these simple guidelines

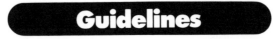

Guidelines

- **Know your meal plan.** Know how many exchanges you are allowed for each meal and then make selections accordingly. Most menus include soups, appetizers, entrees, breads, salads, and desserts. Use your exchanges wisely.

- **Watch serving sizes.** Be familiar with your usual portion size so you will be able to judge correctly what you should eat. Don't feel you have to eat all the food. In a restaurant it is perfectly acceptable to ask for a "doggie bag." You can save that extra food for lunch the next day. If portion sizes are too large and you don't want to ask for a doggie bag, leave the food. It's more important to keep your diabetes under control than to clean your plate.

- **Ask about foods.** If you are not sure how a dish is prepared, ask the person waiting on you. While you are still learning, it may be wise to select simply prepared foods and avoid rich sauces and casseroles with many ingredients. Consider how the food was prepared—was it broiled, baked, roasted, fried, or breaded? What accompanies the selection—gravy, whipping cream, sour cream?

- **Ask that sauces and dressings be served separately.** Request that sauces and dressings be served on the side so you can control the amounts. That way you can eat only small quantities of fats such as salad dressings, butter or margarine, gravies, sauces, whipped cream, and sour cream.

- **Plan ahead.** You can move one meat exchange and all the fat exchanges you can spare from another time of day to your meal out. It is a good idea to save as many fat exchanges as you can, because meals out usually contain more fat than meals at home.

- **Use interchanges.** Know which food groups can be exchanged for other food groups. The easiest interchange is between the fruit and starch/bread lists:

1 fruit exchange = 1 starch/bread exchange

Using interchanges, if fruit is not available, you can have a starch/bread serving instead. If you wish more fruit than is allowed on your meal plan, use a starch bread exchange.

Milk can also be interchanged with items from the starch/bread and meat lists:

1 nonfat milk exchange = 1 starch/bread exchange +
1 lean meat exchange

or

1 nonfat milk exchange +
1 fat exchange = 1 starch/bread exchange +
1 medium fat meat exchange

This is helpful when you would prefer a larger serving of meat and a starch/bread item instead of milk.

- **Adjust meal times.** Insulin-dependent people must remember to eat on schedule. If a meal is delayed by one hour, have a fruit or starch/bread exchange from your meal plan at the normally scheduled meal time. If the meal is delayed for longer than one and one-half hours, move a snack to the meal time and have the meal at snack time. For example, if you will be eating dinner out at 8:30 and your dinner hour is normally 6:00, have the equivalent of your evening snack at 6:00 and then dinner at 8:30.

If you normally take insulin before dinner, as well as in the morning, you have two options: 1) You can take your insulin at the usual time, have your snack, and then dinner later. 2) If dinner is not delayed more than one and one-half hours, you can wait, take your insulin before the meal, and then have the snack before bedtime.

Making these changes will probably affect your blood glucose readings because you may be testing closer to the large meal than you normally do.

- **Use diet and low calorie products when available.** Some restaurants now have diet syrups, jams, and jellies. These items may not appear on the menu but may be available if you request them.

- **Watch preparation.** How foods are cooked affects their exchange value. For example, breaded and deep fat fried foods such as chicken and shrimp contain an additional starch/bread exchange as well as 1 or 2 additional fat exchanges per serving. Meat as listed on a menu refers to the portion size before cooking. It will lose about one-fourth of its size in cooking. For instance, an 8 ounce steak is approximately 6, not 8, meat exchanges.

- **Oops!** Lastly, if you feel you have indeed "blown it," remember the one thing you can do is exercise! Granted, it takes a lot of exercise, but dancing, an exercise bike, or a brisk walk can help. Often individuals will ask about taking extra regular insulin. If you thought you would do okay and then find you "blew it", taking extra regular insulin after the fact really won't help much. By the time you get home, take the extra insulin, and wait for it to peak (remember regular insulin has its peak effect in two to four hours), your food will be all digested. The time to take extra regular insulin is before a meal—not after. Also, it should only be one or two extra units—not five or ten as many individuals want to add. Exercise usually is the better choice.

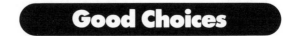

Good Choices

Appetizers:	Tomato juice and other vegetable juices, fruit juice, clear broth, bouillon, consomme, raw vegetables, fresh fruit cocktail.
Meat, Fish, Poultry:	Roasted, baked, or broiled meat, fish, poultry, or seafood.
	Ask that gravy or sauces be omitted and trim excess fat from meats. Be aware that some restaurants will add fat to meat or fish before broiling. If the serving exceeds your portion size remember the doggie bag. Filet mignon or a shish kabob is a good choice when ordering beef: the portion size is reasonable and the meat is lean. Broiled quarter-pound hamburgers, without the high fat sauces, are about 3 meat exchanges and the bun is 2 starch/bread exchanges.
Potatoes:	Mashed, baked, broiled, or steamed potatoes, rice, or noodles.
	Ask for butter, margarine or sour cream "on the side" so you can govern the portion used.
Salads:	Vegetable or fresh fruit salads.
	Use a lemon wedge, vinegar, or known amount of dressing. (One tablespoon of regular dressing equals 1 fat exchange; 2 to 3 tablespoons of a low-calorie or reduced-calorie dressing equals 1 fat exchange.)

Vegetables:	Stewed, steamed, boiled, or broiled.
	If buttered, allow 1 fat exchange for each 1/2 cup serving.
Fruit:	Fresh fruit, fresh fruit salad, or fruit juices.
Breads:	Order breads that are not frosted or glazed.
	For variety, substitute hard or soft dinner rolls, French bread (3″ slice), plain muffin, biscuits, crackers, popovers. Other substitutes for one bread exchange: two 8″ long bread sticks, 4 melba toast rectangles or 8 rounds, 4 Ry-Krisp, 1/2 bagel or English muffin, 1/2 hamburger or hot dog bun (1 if small or about 1 oz.).
Desserts:	Fresh fruit, plain ice cream or sherbet, sponge cake, or angel food cake.
Fats:	Margarine, butter, salad dressing, sour cream. Be careful of amounts!
Beverages:	Coffee, tea, skim milk, diet pop.

If you choose other foods, you will be eating hidden fat, sugar, and calories.

In summary, think about the following guidelines:

1. Of primary importance is familiarity with your meal plan.

2. Be familiar with the restaurant where you will be eating and some of the choices available to you. In general, the more variety and number of choices there are on a menu, the more apt you are to find something that will fit into your meal plan.

3. Decide ahead of time what you plan to order. Many persons have had the experience of going through a cafeteria or buffet and ending up with much more food than they can actually eat. Everything "looks so good" it's hard to pass up! If you have decided ahead of time what you plan to select, you will be less likely to be swayed by all the other choices available to you!

4. Order first at a restaurant. Have you noticed how often the rest of the table orders what the first person chooses? Be the trend setter by ordering first. You won't be as apt to be influenced by what the others order and better yet, they will probably follow your example—and all will benefit!

Chapter Twenty-One
THE FAST FOOD
PHENOMENOM

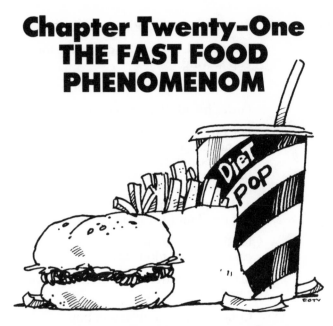

Today in the United States, 200 customers order one or more hamburgers every second! From 1970 to 1980, the number of fast-food restaurants increased from 30,000 to 140,000. Sales in 1970 were $6.5 billion, in 1980, $23 billion, and in 1986, $34 billion. This is approximately 40 percent of total annual sales for all U.S. restaurants, or $2 of every $5 spent in restaurants. U.S. consumers spend an average of $200 a year on fast foods.

Fast-food restaurants usually offer standardized items at reasonable prices with quick service in a clean, well-lit place. Each restaurant tends to be limited to a one-food theme, such as hamburger, fried chicken, roast beef, pizza, fried fish and chips or Mexican food, with some accompaniments and beverages. Fast food menus often contain items that, if properly selected, do comprise meals adequate in protein and some vitamins and minerals. However, many of the food items are very high in calories. Fat (especially saturated fat and cholesterol) and sugar supply a good deal of the calories without providing any other nutrients. Many menu items also contain large amounts of sodium (salt).

The good news is that today many fast-food restaurants offer salad bars, soups, baked potatoes, and sugar-free soft drinks, helping their customers to limit calories, sodium, and fat in a meal. A salad or a baked potato adds complex carbohydrates and fiber, which are missing from traditional fast foods. And if you go easy on the dressings, butter or margarine, and toppings your meal will contain very little fat or sugar. A meal of salad, diet soda and a plain hamburger (without cheese or mayonnaise-based sauce) is fairly low in calories (450 calories).

How to Avoid the Pitfalls

For most people, an occasional meal at a fast-food restaurant will not upset an otherwise well-balanced diet. People who eat fast foods regularly, however, need to choose menu selections with more care.

Calories. The greatest nutritional problem with typical fast food is the number of calories. A lunch of a quarter-pound burger, fries, and a shake contains about 1,150 calories, which is more than most home-prepared dinners. This lunch also contains about 1,080 milligrams of sodium (equal to 1/2 teaspoon of salt) and 45 grams of fat (5 teaspoons) with fat contributing 43 percent of the calories. This is about 40 percent of the number of daily calories needed to maintain the weight of a 165-pound man, and 60 percent of that needed by a 128-pound woman. For someone on a diet, 1,150 calories is a good portion of an entire day's allowance. Teenage boys, on the other hand, can consume such high calorie meals, but the rest of the population can't afford so much of one day's caloric allotment in one meal. And even teenagers need to avoid high fat diets, which can contribute to heart and blood vessel problems later in life.

The key to reducing calories is to buy small and eat only at meal times. The average calorie count of a fast-food meal is 685, which is not outrageously high. However, many people buy fast-food items as snacks rather than meals; the average calorie count for a so-called snack is 427. Added to regular meals, that many calories can put individuals well over their calorie requirements.

Deep-fried foods contain more fat than grilled or broiled foods. If you do order fried foods, discard the breading and avoid the "extra crispy" version. Fried foods, such as chicken, fish, pie, and French fries contain as much as 40 to 60 percent fat. Look for broiled or baked fish and season with lemon juice instead of butter or tartar sauce. Look for baked or broiled chicken as well, hold the sauces, and discard the breading.

Processed meats are high in fat, so avoid bacon on your burger, pepperoni on pizza, and sausage on a biscuit. A plain pizza topped with vegetables instead of meat is much lower in fat. Two slices of a 16-inch cheese pizza contains 400 calories, only 18 percent of which are from fat. Order pizza with mushrooms, green pepper, and onions. When you add pepperoni, sausage, anchovies, or extra cheese, you add unnecessary fat, sodium, and calories.

Sodium. To lower sodium consumption, order foods without condiments. One tablespoon of ketchup contains 150 mg. of sodium, and 1 tablespoon of mustard contains about 180 mg. Together, they make up nearly 1/5 of your total daily salt allotment. To cut down on salt, hold pickles, ketchup, and special sauces.

Fiber. Beans are one of the best sources of fiber; baked beans, chili with beans, and refried beans all add fiber to your meal. At the salad bar, choose kidney beans, garbanzo beans, and fruit to add fiber. Baked potatoes with skin are another good choice for fiber; however, ordering only the skins usually means deep-fat fried skins with salty, fatty toppings.

Whenever possible, order whole grain buns, but be wary of "wheat" bread products containing caramel coloring to make them look dark. They are not rich in whole grains. You should see flecks of fiber in your whole-wheat bread products.

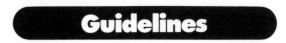

Guidelines

People with diabetes will at times find it convenient or necessary to use fast foods. When you do, the following guidelines can help you make wise decisions.

Know your meal plan. You will need to choose foods that fit into your available exchanges for meals or snacks.

Know the nutritional value of fast-food items. Fast-food chains may be easier to predict than some expensive gourmet restaurants. Studies of the leading chains show remarkable uniformity in portion size and nutritional value of their food.

Avoid the high-fat, high-saturated fat item. Avoid large orders of high-fat foods, such as a double-cheeseburger. Instead, settle for a more moderate-sized burger, such as a plain quarter pounder. Beware of the high-fat, mayonnaise-based sauces added to hamburgers, as well as items such as French fries cooked in saturated fat. Sources of hidden fats and sugars are shakes, fries, apple pies, and soft drinks.

Go easy on salt. Many fast foods are extremely high in salt. Additional items that contain a lot of salt are ketchup, pickles, mustard, tartar sauce, salad dressing, and other condiments.

IN ADDITION, BEWARE OF

- **Croissant sandwiches.** One croissant averages 200 to 250 calories (2 breads, 2 fat exchanges) compared to one whole-grain bun with 135 calories (1½ bread exchanges). Croissant sandwiches average 400 to 600 calories compared to 350 calories for a roast beef sandwich or 285 calories for a pita pocket sandwich.

- **Stuffed potatoes.** A plain baked potato averages 200 to 250 calories (3 breads) with only 2 grams of fat and little sodium. But add bacon and cheese and the calories total 590 and fat soars to 30 to 40 grams (6 to 8 teaspoons). The sodium also skyrockets from 60 to 1,180 milligrams (equal to 1/2 teaspoon of salt). A deluxe superstuffed baked potato with sour cream, butter, bacon, and cheese has 640 calories and 6 teaspoons of fat.

- **Batter-fried chicken and fish.** Chicken and fish normally have a low fat content and relatively few calories, but not when breaded or fried as they usually are in fast-food restaurants. A fried fish sandwich, milkshake and french fries total 935 calories, 1,070 milligrams of sodium, and 42 grams of fat (40 percent of the calories). Chicken sandwiches average 500 to 700 calories (3 bread, 3 to 4 lean meats, and 4 to 6½ fat exchanges). A fish filet sandwich has 450 to 500 calories (2 breads, 2 lean meats, 4 fat exchanges).

- **Large hamburgers with all the cheese and other toppings.** They average 525 to 820 calories.

- **Breakfast biscuits.** They "start your day" with 500 to 700 calories, 30 to 35 grams of fat and more than 1,000 mg. of sodium. A sausage and egg croissant contains 645 milligrams of cholesterol—more than double the recommended amount of 300 milligrams a day. Instead, by ordering a scrambled egg with an English muffin your calories are 366, 17 grams of fat, 515 mg. of sodium. This is still a substantial breakfast but with less fat, sodium and calories.

- **Super hot dogs with cheese.** They have 8 teaspoons of fat along with 1,605 milligrams of sodium. Add a large malt with 1,060 calories—estimated to contain 25 teaspoons of sugar—and you are in trouble. Stick to the single hamburger with lettuce and tomato, small ice cream cone, and diet soda pop.

Good Choices

An occasional meal at a fast-food restaurant will not upset an otherwise well-balanced diet. People who eat fast foods regularly, however, need to make menu selections with more care.

For a fast but healthy breakfast, try a whole grain English muffin or plain toast with a small amount of butter, low fat milk, and fruit or fruit juice. A surprisingly good option is pancakes without butter. They have less fat than croissants and are relatively cholesterol free. Bring with you and use diet jam, jelly, or syrup.

For lunch, a sandwich with lean meats—roast beef, turkey, or ham—and whole-grain bread can be a good choice. Ask them to hold the butter, or margarine, or mayo. Roast beef sandwiches can be better than hamburgers—even the fattest roast beef sandwich is leaner than the leanest hamburger. Avoid anything labeled big, deluxe, or whopper. The smallest hamburger and sandwich will be the lowest in calories and fat. Buy small—avoid double and triple sandwiches. Hold condiments such as tartar sauce, mayonnaise, bacon, and cheese to further reduce the fat and calories. A roasted chicken breast sandwich (if you can find it) is a wonderful choice. It will be both lower in fat and lower in calories (254) than other menu items.

A salad bar is a healthful alternative to high-fat sandwiches. A large salad containing a variety of vegetables, 1/2 cup of cottage cheese, and reduced-calorie salad dressing has less than 250 calories. However, by adding just 1 tablespoon of regular dressing, some bacon bits, and 1/4 cup macaroni or potato salad, you increase the calorie level to 500. If you add cole slaw (1/2 cup, 90 calories), sunflower seeds and raisins (1/4 cup, 180 calories), you quickly add extra calories.

An average fast-food salad with 2 cups lettuce and assorted raw vegetables will average around 80 to 100 calories. Count this as one starch/bread exchange. It could also be counted as 3 vegetable exchanges, but meal plans rarely call for 3 vegetables. Use diet salad dressings. Carry your own diet salad dressing if necessary.

As to accompaniments, save calories and sugar by drinking non-caloric beverages. Skip fast-food desserts; instead satisfy yourself by bringing fresh fruit from home. Try eating your "dessert" fruit first; it is a creative way to curb your appetite and avoid overeating.

And finally, make wise choices. If you go with fast foods for one meal, try to balance this with the rest of your day's choices.

The following list will give you an idea of some fast food choices that might fit into your meal. For more complete information on fast-food restaurants and the nutritive value and exchanges of the foods they serve, see **Fast Food Facts.**

Exchange List

FAST FOOD

Food	Quantity	Calories	Exchanges
Burger King, Burger Chef, **McDonalds, Hardees**			
Hamburger	1	240-275	2 starch/bread 2 med. fat meat

Food	Quantity	Calories	Exchanges
Cheeseburger	1	280-320	2 starch/bread 2 med. fat meat 1 fat
Quarter Pounder	1	430	2 starch/bread 3 med. fat meat 1 fat
French fries	Regular	230	1½ starch/bread 2 fat
Salad with reduced-calorie dressing	1	45	1 vegetable

Dairy Queen

Food	Quantity	Calories	Exchanges
Hamburger	1	360	2 starch/bread 2 med. fat meat 1 fat
Hamburger with cheese	1	410	2 starch/bread 3 med. fat meat 1 fat
French Fries	Regular	200	1½ starch/bread 2 fat
Hot Dog	1	280	1½ starch/bread 1 med. fat meat 2 fat
Hot Dog with chili	1	320	1½ starch/bread 1 med. fat meat 2 fat

For Occasional Use

Food	Quantity	Calories	Exchanges
Frozen dessert	4 oz.	180	2 starch/bread 1 fat
Cone	Regular	240	2½ starch/bread 1 fat
"DQ" sandwich	1	140	1½ starch/bread 1 fat

Wendy's

Food	Quantity	Calories	Exchanges
Hamburger	1	350	2 starch/bread 3 med. fat meat
Chili	Regular	240	1½ starch/bread 2 med. fat meat
Fish fillet	1	210	1 starch/bread 2 med. fat meat

Food	Quantity	Calories	Exchanges
Taco salad	1	430	3 starch/bread 2 med. fat meat 2 fat
Pick up window salad	1	110	1 vegetable 1 fat
Arby's or Rax			
Junior Roast Beef	1	220	1½ starch/bread 1½ med. fat meat
Regular Roast Beef	1	350-370	2 starch/bread 2 med. fat meat 1 fat
Ham 'n Cheese Sandwich	1	350	2 starch/bread 3 med. fat meat
Turkey	1	375	2 starch/bread 3 med. fat meat
Baked potato, plain	1	290	4 starch/bread
Tossed salad with low-calorie dressing	1	60	1 vegetable
Kentucky Fried Chicken **Original Recipe**			
Center Breast	1	60	1/2 starch/bread 3 med. fat meat
Drumstick	1	150	2 med. fat meat
Thigh	1	280	1/2 starch/bread 2 med. fat meat 2 fat
Wing	1	180	1/2 starch/bread 1½ med. fat meat 1 fat
Mashed potato with gravy	1	60	1 starch/bread
Corn-on-the-cob	1	175	2 starch/bread
Baked beans	1	105	1 starch/bread
Cole slaw	1	105	2 vegetable **or** 1 starch/bread 1 fat
Dominos Pizza			
Cheese pizza, 12" pie	2 slices	340	3 starch/bread 1 med. fat meat 1 vegetable

Food	Quantity	Calories	Exchanges
Pepperoni, 12″ pie	2 slices	380	3 starch/bread 2 med. fat meat 1 vegetable
Shakey's			
Thin cheese, 13″ pie	1/10	140	1 starch/bread 1 med. fat meat
Thin pepperoni, 13″ pie	1/10	185	1 starch/bread 2 med. fat meat
Taco Bell, Zantigo			
Bean Burrito	1	360	3½ starch/bread 1 med. fat meat 1 fat
Beef Burrito	1	415-460	2½ starch/bread 2 med. fat meat 1 fat
Taco	1	185-200	1 starch/bread 1-2 lean meat 1 fat
Taco Salad*	1	950	4 starch/bread 3 med. fat meat 9 fat
Tostada	1	240	2 starch/bread 1 med. fat meat 1 fat
Red Lobster			
Lunch portion of fish (Dinner portion twice as large)	5 oz.	130-190	3 lean meat
Maine Lobster	1 tail	260	5 lean meat
Chicken Breast	4 oz.	120	3 lean meat

*Notice high calorie and fat content!

Chapter Twenty-Two
IF ALCOHOL IS USED

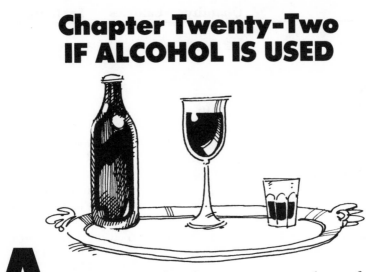

Alcoholic beverages have become an accepted part of our social lives. The decision to use or not use alcoholic beverages must be made by each individual. When making this decision, the individual with diabetes needs to be aware of the effects of alcohol on the body, as well as the effect of alcohol on blood glucose control.

Metabolism of Alcohol

Research has shown how the body deals with alcohol and why it is damaging, particularly to the liver and brain, if taken in excess.

Alcohol is broken down in the liver by specific enzymes at a constant rate. The human body can burn about one ounce of alcohol (7 to 10 grams of pure ethanol alcohol) per hour. Alcohol is a depressant; it slows down brain activity. However, the initial subjective feeling is just the opposite, because it lifts the barriers of self control.

The overall effect of alcohol is to lower blood glucose levels. When you have not eaten for a period of time, your liver becomes depleted of its stored carbohydrate (glycogen). Normally, the liver then converts noncarbohydrate sources, such as protein, into glucose to maintain blood sugar. When the liver is metabolizing alcohol, the formation of glucose from other sources is blocked. Alcohol cannot be converted to glucose. It can only be used for energy or converted to fat. If the calories from alcohol are not used as an immediate energy source, they are stored as fat.

Hypoglycemia can occur even when blood alcohol levels do not exceed the range of mild intoxication and is particularly a problem when food intake has been restricted. Two ounces (20 to 25 grams of pure ethanol alcohol) of alcohol is enough to produce hypoglycemia in a person who has not eaten for several hours. Persons in poor control of their diabetes usually have depleted glycogen stores, so they are at special risk of hypoglycemia.

The metabolism of alcohol does **not** require insulin. In fact, it augments the effects of insulin. Alcohol does not stimulate insulin secretion, but enhances the glucose-lowering action of insulin or other hypoglycemic agents. The presence of alcohol in the blood can prolong the effect of a single injection of insulin.

Large doses of alcohol may cause a small but transient rise in blood glucose, but it is followed a couple of hours later by a fall in blood glucose to below the fasting level. This hyperglycemia occurs later in the course of alcohol ingestion, frequently when the effects of alcohol concentrations are declining. The overall effect of alcohol is a significant reduction of blood glucose levels. A high fat diet and alcohol can also cause an increase in ketones.

Alcohol is a concentrated source of calories, yielding seven calories per gram. For comparison, carbohydrate and protein yield four calories per gram and fat yields nine calories per gram. Alcohol provides energy but no nourishment. One ounce of 86 proof liquor contains about ten grams of alcohol or 70 calories. Sweet wines and beer also contain carbohydrate, so they have additional calories.

When diabetes is well controlled, the blood glucose level is not affected by the moderate use of alcohol consumed shortly before, during or after eating. However, alcohol should be avoided in certain conditions: persons with high triglyceride levels, gastritis, pancreatitis and certain types of kidney and heart diseases. Alcohol also interacts with barbituates, tranquilizers and a number of other drugs.

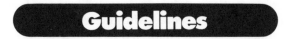

Guidelines

Many individuals with diabetes can include alcohol in their meal plan by following some simple guidelines. These guidelines refer to the occasional use of alcoholic beverages. Approximately two equivalents of alcohol not more than once or twice a week is the recommended amount. If alcohol is used daily, limit the amount and be sure to count the calories in your meal plan.

- **Use alcohol only in moderation.** Sip slowly and make a drink last a long time. Even one drink is enough to give the breath the smell of alcohol. Since symptoms of alcohol intoxication and hypoglycemia are similar, it is easy for other people to mistake the low blood sugar for intoxication and delay necessary treatment.

- **Limit yourself to two equivalents of alcohol per day.** Occasional use of carbohydrate-free alcohol can be an "extra" if used by a normal weight insulin-dependent person whose diabetes is well controlled. If used daily, the energy value of alcohol should be included in your daily meal plan. No food should be omitted because of the possibility of alcohol-induced hypoglycemia. The amount of alcohol contained in each of the following is one equivalent:

  1.5 oz. of a distilled beverage — whiskey, Scotch, rye, vodka, gin, cognac, rum, dry brandy
  4 oz. of dry wine; 2 oz. of dry sherry
  12 oz. of beer, preferably light

- **Count the calories.** Persons with non-insulin-dependent diabetes, for whom weight is a concern, must count the calories from alcohol in their meal plan. Calories are best substituted for fat exchanges — alcohol is metabolized in a manner similar to fat. (Each of the above equivalents is equal to two fat exchanges.)

- **Never drink on an empty stomach.** Avoid hypoglycemia if you are taking insulin, especially when drinking before meals or during times of peak insulin action. Two equivalents of alcohol shortly before a meal or directly after should be safe.

- **Avoid drinks that contain large amounts of sugar.** Liqueurs, sweet wines and sweet mixes (such as tonic, soda pop or fruit juices) are examples of drinks containing sugar. Beer and ale contain malt sugar, which should be substituted for carbohydrate in the meal plan. Light beer is recommended because it has approximately 3 to 6 grams of carbohydrate per can in contrast to regular beer, which has 15 grams of carbohydrate per can. Drink mixes, if used, should be sugar free.

- **Don't let a drink make you careless.** Alcohol can have a relaxing effect and may dull judgment. Be sure meals and snacks are taken on time and selected with the usual care. A too generous intake of alcohol may lead to further dietary indiscretion.

- **Carry identification.** Visible identification that you have diabetes should be carried or worn when drinking away from home.

- **Oral hypoglycemic agents may not mix with alcohol.** In some people, the oral hypoglycemic agents (the sulfonylurea group, especially chlorpropamide) interact with alcohol to produce deep flushing, nausea, quickened heart beat and impaired speech. This set of undesirable symptoms is called the "disulfiram reaction." It occurs in 10 to 30 percent of those using oral hypoglycemic agents. This reaction is rare for individuals who use the second generation of oral hypoglycemics.

Composition of Alcoholic Beverages

Beer and ale are made by fermenting grain mash to malt sugar and ethanol. A 12 ounce can of regular beer contains approximately 15 grams of carbohydrate.

Light beers have less carbohydrate and alcohol than regular beer. They contain 3 to 6 grams of carbohydrate per 12 ounce can.

Distilled spirits are grain mash fermented to 40 percent ethanol. They have a high alcohol content with virtually no carbohydrate.

Liqueurs (or cordials) — have sugar content as high as 50 percent and alcohol concentrations from 20 to 55 percent. They are not recommended for use by individuals with diabetes.

Nonalcoholic — describes nonalcoholic malt beverages with less than 0.5 percent alcohol.

Dry sherries are low in carbohydrate (less than 2 grams).

Sweet sherries, port and muscatel, contain approximately 7 grams of carbohydrate per 2 ounce serving.

Wines are fermented fruit juice. They are dry or sweet depending on whether or not all the sugar has been allowed to change to ethanol. Most wines contain 12 percent ethyl alcohol content; **dry wines** contain .1 to .3 percent carbohydrate; **sweet wines** may have 15 percent or more carbohydrate and are not recommended.

Wine coolers — combination of wine and fruit juice, usually in equal portions, to which carbonation and a sweetener have been added. They have an alcoholic content that ranges from 3 to 7 percent.

De-alcoholized wines are basically fruit juice; 4 ounces contain 7 grams of carbohydrate and 35 calories.

Alcoholic Beverages

Beverage	Serving	Alcohol (gms)	Carbo-hydrate (gms)	Calories	Exchanges For Non-Insulin-Dependent Diabetes
Beer:					
Regular beer	12 oz.	13.0	13.7	151	1 starch/bread 2 fat
Light beer	12 oz.	10.1	6	90	2 fat
Extra light beer	12 oz.	8.1	3.3	70	1½ fat
Near beer	12 oz.	1.5	12.3	60	1 starch/bread
Nonalcoholic beer	11 oz.	.3	9.7	50	1 starch/bread
Distilled spirits:					
86 proof (gin, rum, vodka, whiskey, Scotch)	1½ oz.	15.3	Trace	107	2 fat
Dry brandy or cognac	1 oz.	10.7	Trace	75	1½ fat
Table wines:					
Red or Rosé	4 oz.	11.6	1.0	85	2 fat
Dry white	4 oz.	11.3	.4	80	2 fat
Sweet wine	4 oz.	11.8	4.9	102	1/3 starch/bread 2 fat
Light wine	4 oz.	6.4	1.3	48-58	1 fat
Wine coolers	12 oz.	15.0	22.0	192	1½ fruit, 3 fat
Sparkling wines:					
Champagne	4 oz.	11.9	3.6	98	2 fat
Sweet Kosher wine	4 oz.	11.9	12.0	132	1 starch/bread 2 fat
Appetizer/dessert wines:					
Sherry	2 oz.	9.4	1.5	73	1½ fat
Sweet sherry, port, muscatel	2 oz.	9.4	7.0	94	1/2 starch/bread 1½ fat
Vermouths:					
Dry	3 oz.	12.6	4.2	105	2 fat
Sweet	3 oz.	12.2	13.9	141	1 starch/bread 2 fat

Chapter Twenty-Three
MEAL PLANNING
DURING BRIEF ILLNESS

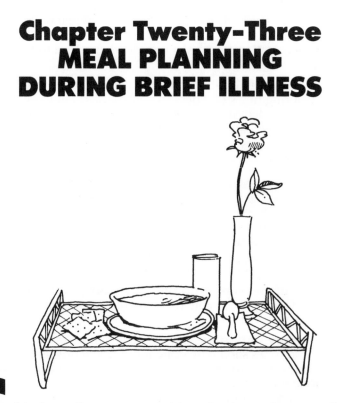

Colds, fever, flu, nausea, vomiting, diarrhea—these are all common illnesses that may cause special problems for people with diabetes.

During illness diabetes control can deteriorate rapidly. Fever, dehydration (the loss of water), infection and the stress of illness can all trigger the release of hormones (sometimes called "stress hormones" or counter-regulatory hormones, such as adrenalin, noradrenalin, glucagon, cortisol, growth hormone) that raise blood glucose causing insulin needs to be increased. Insulin is the main hormone that lowers blood glucose levels.

During stress, such as illness, these "stress" hormones normally provide the brain and muscles with sources of energy by raising the levels of glucose and ketones. In non-diabetics this elevation does not get out of hand because additional insulin is also released, which prevents blood glucose from rising too high. Insulin also prevents the uncontrolled breakdown of fat and excessive build-up of ketones in the blood. For individuals with diabetes, the actions of the "stress hormones" tend to be unchecked or poorly checked because of the lack of effective insulin. When the body does not have the help of sufficient insulin, the ketones build up in the blood and then "spill into the urine" so the body can get rid of them. When present in large amounts in the blood, ketones (which are types of acids) cause ketoacidosis. Ketoacidosis, if untreated, can lead to coma and even death.

Persons with non-insulin-dependent diabetes may need insulin temporarily during times of illness to control blood glucose. Persons with insulin-dependent diabetes must have insulin throughout illness to prevent ketoacidosis. The insulin is needed even if the individual is eating less than usual as a result of nausea and vomiting. In fact, insulin requirements usually increase during illness.

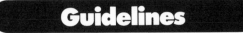

Guidelines

- **Your need for insulin continues,** or may even increase. If in doubt, begin by taking your normal amount of insulin or diabetes pill (oral agent). If you normally don't use regular insulin, have a vial of regular insulin on reserve to use during illness if directed.

- **If you take diabetes pills do not take your pill if you are vomiting.** Once you are able to keep fluids down and begin taking food, take your pill.

- **Testing is very important.** Blood glucose monitoring and urine testing for ketones should be done more frequently. Even with blood glucose monitoring you still need to test urine for ketones. If the blood glucose level is higher than 240 mg./dl., it is especially important to test for ketones.

- **Replace carbohydrates** with liquids or soft foods if you cannot eat your regular foods. At least 50 grams of carbohydrates should be consumed every three to four hours. It is important to use small, frequent feedings. This is necessary to provide some readily available sugar so the body won't have to burn fat and to prevent blood glucose levels from dropping too rapidly.

- **Drink fluids and take aspirin** — the usual advice during illness — is also helpful for persons with diabetes. Fluids are important to prevent dehydration, and the aspirin reduces fever and controls secretion of the stress-produced hormones. Children should use an aspirin substitute such as Tylenol. Body fluids and minerals are rapidly depleted during illness. Water, clear broth, tea and other fluids should be taken frequently.

The above steps apply to mild, short-term (approximately one day) illnesses. Remember that acidosis and dehydration can develop very rapidly, especially in children. You should contact your health care providers if:

- **You are unable to eat solid foods for more than one day or you are unable to keep replacement foods down.**

- **You are spilling ketones in your urine.**

The following foods contain concentrated sugar and are easily tolerated by most people during a brief illness. Remember — you want to take in about 50 grams of carbohydrate every three to four hours or for each missed meal. This should be done in small, frequent feedings.

To replace **10 grams of carbohydrate**, use any of the following foods in the amount indicated.

Food	Quantity
Carbonated beverage containing sugar (ginger ale, Coca-Cola, Pepsi-Cola)*	1/2 cup (4 oz.)
Popsicle	1/2 twin bar
Corn syrup or honey	2 tsp.
Granulated sugar	2½ tsp. or 5 small sugar cubes
Sweetened gelatin (Jell-O)	1/4 cup
Coke syrup	1 Tbsp. (1.2 oz.)

To replace **15 grams of carbohydrate**, use any of the following foods in the amount indicated.

Food	Quantity
Ice cream	1/2 cup
Cooked cereal	1/2 cup
Sherbet	1/4 cup
Jell-O	1/3 cup
Broth based soups, reconstituted with water	1 cup
Cream soups	1 cup
Carbonated beverage containing sugar (ginger ale, Coca-Cola, Pepsi-Cola)*	3/4 cup (6 oz.)
Orange or grapefruit juice	1/2 cup
Grape juice	1/3 cup

*Soda pop opened and left at room temperature for a few minutes to allow for "decarbonation" will usually be better tolerated.

Food	Quantity
Popsicles	1 pop
Milk shake	1/4 cup
Milk	1¼ cups (10 oz.)
Eggnog, commercial	1/2 cup
Tapioca pudding	1/3 cup
Custard	1/2 cup
Yogurt, plain	1 cup
Toast	1 slice
Saltine crackers	6

Chapter Twenty-Four
EXERCISE CAUTION
WHEN EXERCISING

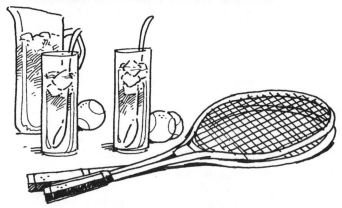

Exercise can be beneficial to everyone's health. In fact, it may have some added benefits for you if you have diabetes. The person with diabetes will experience the same benefits and enjoyment everyone else gains from exercise: increased muscle strength and endurance and more efficient heart and lungs. Psychologically, exercise helps you cope with stress. You build self-confidence and improve your self-image, especially when you discover that your "nonathletic" picture of yourself may be incorrect. Of course, exercise is important for maintaining appropriate body weight. Fat stores decrease as you increase the amount of muscle that develops with exercise.

Diabetes should not be a reason to avoid physical activity. In addition to the above benefits, persons with diabetes can experience some added benefits from exercise: Regular exercise increases sensitivity to insulin and therefore reduces insulin requirements. Also, the body's ability to handle glucose improves.

Physical activity can help to reverse the resistance to insulin that occurs as a result of obesity. Further, exercise improves risk factors related to heart disease. This includes a lowering of blood cholesterol and triglycerides and an increase in high density cholesterol, the type of cholesterol that protects against heart disease. Exercise also lowers blood pressure.

Before beginning an exercise program it is important to get your doctor's approval—especially if you are over age 30 or have had diabetes for ten years or more. Problems such as eye, kidney, or nerve damage may be worsened by inappropriate or strenuous exercise. Nerve damage can blunt or block the body's signals of pain or discomfort from exercise, leading to serious damage before you notice it. Foot problems can develop if proper precautions are not taken.

Along with the benefits, exercise poses some risks to persons with diabetes. You need to know how to prevent hypoglycemia (low blood glucose) and to be aware of the effects of exercising with hyperglycemia (too high blood glucose).

Hypoglycemia

A major function of insulin is to block production of glucose by the liver. In persons who do not have diabetes, insulin levels decrease during exercise. When insulin levels go down, the liver speeds up glucose production so blood glucose levels stay in the normal range. This occurs in spite of the fact that exercising can increase glucose use twenty-fold above non-exercising needs.

However, if you require injected insulin your body cannot decrease the level of circulating insulin when you begin to exercise. When serum insulin remains elevated, production of glucose by the liver is inhibited. As a result your body uses what glucose is available, but there is no increase in glucose production to meet the added needs of the exercising muscle. Hypoglycemia can result.

Hypoglycemia can occur during exercise—usually when you exercise for longer than an hour, but it can also occur for as long as 24 hours after strenuous or prolonged exercise. After you finish exercising your body has to replace the stored carbohydrate (glycogen) you used during exercise. Therefore blood glucose levels can continue to drop after exercise.

Hypoglycemia can be prevented by increasing food before and/ or after exercise or by reducing the dosage of insulin acting during the time of activity. See page 143 for guidelines on how to begin doing this.

Monitoring of blood glucose levels before, during, and after exercise is the single greatest tool for planning an appropriate dosage of insulin as well as food intake to prevent hypoglycemia.

Hyperglycemia

Although the major concern usually is low blood glucose levels as a consequence of exercise, there are times when exercise can raise blood glucose levels. You will remember that one of the primary roles of insulin is to allow the use of glucose by muscles. With exercise you need less insulin to allow this to happen, but you do need some insulin.

Therefore if you begin exercise with an insulin deficiency—

such as occurs with uncontrolled diabetes—blood glucose levels and ketones can rise with exercise. How does this happen? When blood glucose is elevated (generally greater than 250 to 300 mg./dl.) as a result of insufficient insulin (poor control), exercise cannot increase glucose uptake by the muscle since this requires insulin. The exercising muscles still need glucose and will send a message to the liver to produce or release stored carbohydrate. As a result, glucose production will be stimulated, resulting in a further rise in blood glucose during exercise. There can also be an increase in blood ketone levels if too much fat is being released as a response to the decreased levels of insulin in the blood. The breakdown of fat to ketones exceeds the ability of muscles to use them.

If you begin exercise when your blood glucose level is greater than 250 to 300 mg./dl., you may find that exercise does not decrease these high glucose levels. In fact, glucose may increase even more, and there can also be an accumulation of ketones. Activity is not a replacement for insulin. You need adequate amounts of insulin available for the muscles to use glucose during exercise. However, with mild to moderate hyperglycemia—blood glucose levels under 250 to 300 mg./dl.—moderate exercise will result in a desirable reduction of blood glucose levels.

General Recommendations for Safe Exercise for Persons Taking Injected Insulin

Although studies have not shown that exercise is beneficial in the overall control of blood glucose levels—in fact often blood glucose levels are harder to control with exercise—the overall goal is to allow persons with diabetes to begin and/or continue to exercise safely and enjoy the benefits of that exercise. For most people, the benefits of exercise far exceed the risks.

You will be your own best teacher when making decisions about blood glucose control during exercise. Blood glucose monitoring is your most effective tool for deciding when and how much to increase food intake or how to reduce insulin dosage appropriately.

Ideally, you would exercise at approximately the same time each day and at the same level of intensity. For practical reasons this may not be possible.

In general, persons with diabetes tend to overeat before exercise, possibly because of over-cautiousness and concern about hypoglycemia or through a belief that exercise will alleviate the high blood glucose level resulting from overeating.

Six general precautions that need to be taken when planning an exercise program are:

1. Be sure you are in good control of your diabetes. The effect of

exercise will depend on the availability of insulin to muscle cells.

2. Be aware of the peak times of insulin action and the excessive lowering of blood glucose levels that exercise may have at these times. Regular insulin peaks in three to four hours; Lente or NPH in eight to ten hours. An ideal time for exercise is following a meal, especially after breakfast since blood glucose levels tend to be the highest during the morning hours. If you do exercise when insulin is at its peak time of action be sure to plan for appropriate increase in carbohydrates.

3. Be aware that exercise may accelerate the rate of insulin absorption from the injected site. This is of particular concern if you exercise immediately after doing your injection. If 40 minutes or more have elapsed between the regular insulin injection and the start of exercise, more than half of the injected insulin will be mobilized from the injection site. Likewise intermediate-acting insulin absorption remains unaffected when exercise is begun two and one-half hours after the injection. Thus you only need to rotate the sites of insulin injection to parts of the body that are not involved in the physical activity, when exercise is begun immediately after an insulin injection. In that case, inject into a non-exercising area, such as the abdomen, which will minimize the effect of exercise on insulin absorption.

4. Food intake may need to be increased to accommodate activity or exercise. Regular periods of activity will be planned for in your meal plan. Well-trained individuals who regularly exercise will usually need less additional food than people who exercise only occasionally. The best way to determine how much extra food is needed is to monitor your blood glucose before, during and after exercise, especially in the planning stages.

Extra food eaten before exercise should be in addition to your regular meal plan. In general 10 to 15 grams of carbohydrate—one fruit or starch/bread exchange—should be eaten before an hour of moderate exercise. This is of particular importance if your blood glucose levels have been in the normal range. Moderate exercise includes tennis, swimming, jogging, cycling, or gardening. For more strenuous activity, 30 to 50 grams of carbohydrate—one-half a meat sandwich with one milk or fruit exchange—may be needed. Football, hockey, racketball, basketball, strenuous cycling or swimming, or shoveling heavy snow are examples of strenuous activity. Mild exercise, such as walking a half mile, will probably not require any extra food.

The effect of exercise on blood glucose levels varies greatly. Everyone exercises at different intensities and uses insulin and food differently. The guidelines given in the Food Adjustments for Exercise table are only recommendations. They can help you to plan food for exercise and to make food changes based on your own blood glucose level. But it's still important for you to monitor your blood glucose level and adapt these guidelines to your own needs. Along with food intake, exercisers must remember the need for increased fluid intake. Individuals whose diabetes is poorly controlled are particularly at risk for dehydration when exercising on warm days.

5. Blood glucose levels can continue to decrease after exercise. The body may need up to 24 hours to replace the stored carbohydrate (glycogen) used during exercise. By monitoring blood glucose levels at one or two intervals after strenuous exercise, you can assess how you respond to the blood glucose lowering effects of exercise.

6. Be sure to carry adequate identification with you and a source of readily available carbohydrate as well.

In summary, if the proper precautions are taken, the effect of exercise on a well-controlled insulin-user will be to increase glucose uptake in the exercising muscle, resulting in a lowering of blood glucose levels. It will also increase the body's sensitivity to insulin. Excessive fall of blood glucose levels can be avoided by avoiding peak insulin times, and eating additional carbohydrate.

The body's response to exercise depends on insulin being available. So make sure your diabetes is under good control before beginning an exercise session. In addition, monitor blood glucose levels before and after exercise.

Food Adjustments for Exercise

Type of Exercise and Examples:	If Blood Sugar is:	Increase Food Intake by:	Suggested Food:
Exercise of short duration or of moderate intensity	less than 80 to 100 mg./dl.	10 to 15 gms. of carbohydrate	1 fruit **or** 1 starch/bread exchange
	100 mg./dl. or above	not necessary to increase food	

Examples:
Walking a half mile or leisurely biking for one mile

Type of Exercise and Examples:	If Blood Sugar Is:	Increase Food Intake By:	Suggested Food:
Exercise of Moderate intensity	less than 80 to 100 mg./dl.	25 to 50 gms. of carbohydrate before exercise, then 10 to 15 gms. per hour of exercise, if necessary	1/2 meat sandwich with milk **or** fruit exchange
Examples: Tennis, swimming, jogging, leisure cycling, gardening golfing or vacuuming for one hour	80 to 170 mg./dl.	10 to 15 gms. of carbohydrate	1 fruit **or** 1 starch/bread exchange
	180-300 mg./dl. *250*	not necessary to increase food	
	300 mg./dl. or greater *250*	don't begin exercise until blood sugar is under better control	
Strenuous activity or exercise	less than 80 to 100 mg./dl.	50 gms. of carbohydrate, monitor blood sugars carefully	1 meat sandwich (2 slices of bread) with a milk and a fruit exchange
Examples: Football, hockey, racquetball or basketball games; strenuous cycling or swimming; shoveling heavy snow for one hour	180 to 300 mg./dl. *250*	10 to 15 gms. of carbohydrate per hour of exercise	1 fruit or 1 starch/bread exchange
	300 mg./dl. or greater *250*	don't begin exercise until blood sugar is under better control	

Guidelines

When exercising strenuously over an extended period of time—all morning, all afternoon or all day—begin to adjust insulin by using the following guideline:

Decrease insulin acting during the exercise time by 10 percent of the total insulin dose.

Example:
Insulin dose: 4 Regular 24 NPH before breakfast
2 Regular 6 NPH before evening meal

Total dose = units (4 + 2 + 24 + 6 = 36)
10 percent of total dose = 3.6 units (36 x .10) or 4 units

Rapid-acting insulin (Regular) acts during the morning hours. For cross-country skiing all morning, decrease the a.m. rapid-acting by 10 percent of the total insulin dose. The morning insulin would be 0 Regular (4 − 4) and 24 NPH.

Intermediate-acting insulin (NPH, Lente) taken before breakfast will act during the afternoon hours. For canoeing all afternoon, the morning insulin would be 4 Regular and 20 NPH (24 − 4).

For an activity lasting the entire day, such as downhill skiing or backpacking, both the Regular and NPH would be decreased so the morning insulin would be 0 Regular (4 − 4) and 20 NPH (24 − 4)

Athletes with Insulin-Dependent Diabetes

Individuals with IDDM are often involved in strenuous or competitive activities such as all day athletic events, marathon running, long distance cycling, etc., and may find the following guidelines helpful. An athlete's response to exertion is highly individual and will differ based on many factors during training and competition. Therefore, only approximate guidelines can be given. Keeping records of all variables and their effects during training is the best way for an individual to determine insulin adjustments and fluid and food intake to maximize performance on days of competition.

1. Choose a time to train when blood glucose is above fasting, perhaps an hour or two after a meal.

2. Athletes may require a source of carbohydrate during exercise of long duration, such as a long run or athletic event lasting several hours. Fruit juice can be a good source of carbohydrate and fluid but should be diluted with water (1 part juice to 3 parts water) so it can be absorbed more quickly. Athletes should try to consume 10 to 15 grams of carbohydrate every hour during a long event. Do not wait for symptoms of hypoglycemia to develop; loss of consciousness is not only embarrassing but may go unnoticed or be misunderstood by others during the excitement of an athletic event.

3. During breaks in long lasting athletic events, watery fruits such as oranges, apples, peaches, plums, and pears can help prevent low blood glucose without providing too much sugar. They are approximately 85 percent water so they provide fluids as well.

4. Athletes should carry some form of carbohydrate-containing foods with them in case hypoglycemia does occur. Change for a telephone call or vending machine can also be useful. Informing

teammates and coaches about diabetes and what to do in an emergency is also important.

5. Drink plenty of fluids before, during, and after practice or events. Athletes with IDDM often become so preoccupied with replacing carbohydrate that they forget the most important nutrient needed during regular exercise: Water. For every one pound of weight loss during exercise, 2 cups of fluids are needed for replacement.

6. Athletes with diabetes should not practice carboyhydrate loading, especially regimens that include a period of carbohydrate restriction. Adjusting insulin dosages under these circumstances is just too difficult.

Exercise Benefits for Persons With Non-insulin-dependent Diabetes

Lifestyle changes that include a combination of improved nutrition, safe and enjoyable exercise, weight-loss, and blood glucose monitoring have been shown to be the best means to begin management of NIDDM.

Exercise can assist in improving control of blood glucose. How? Persons with NIDDM are frequently overweight and insulin resistant. Exercise can make the body more sensitive to the actions of insulin and the help overcome this insulin resistance. However, the benefits of exercise on blood glucose levels are short-lived, and exercise must be done on a regular basis for it to help improve blood glucose control. Food intake usually needs to be restricted as well.

If you use insulin or a diabetes pill (oral hypoglycemic agent) the dosage can usually be reduced and in some cases even eventually eliminated as a result of weight control and regular exercise. If you use insulin or an oral agent to help control blood glucose levels you must be aware of the precautions listed in the previous section. However, since your body is still producing some insulin, your blood glucose levels will not be as unstable with exercise as in the person whose pancreas is not producing any insulin.

Exercise also decreases cholesterol and triglyceride levels and increases HDL cholesterol (the "good" cholesterol, a protective factor for coronary heart disease). These improvements occur even in the absence of significant weight loss. Heart disease is a major concern in diabetes, and exercise is one important way of reducing this threat.

Exercise can also be a way to burn up excess calories and to help with weight loss. There are about 3500 calories stored in one pound of body fat, so to lose one pound of fat you must (1) reduce your calorie intake by 3500 calories, (2) increase your activity level by 3500 calories, or (3) do both. Decreasing your calorie intake by

500 calories a day and adding 250 calories of activity gives you a deficit of 5250 calories in one week—a loss of 1½ pounds of fat.

The Using Up Calories table will give you some idea of how much exercise you need to do to burn 250 calories and the number of calories burned in 1 hour of various activities. As you can see, it takes a significant amount of exercise to lose weight by exercise alone—watch what you eat!

A regular exercise program also increases your resting metabolic rate (the number of calories your body burns when at complete rest). Furthermore, the body converts more of the calories eaten into heat instead of fat in people who exercise regularly. These beneficial effects extend well beyond the actual exercise period.

With exercise there will be an increase in lean body mass (muscle), which may result initially in a small increase in body weight since muscle tissue is heavier than fat tissue. In fact, with exercise you may not notice any weight loss although your clothes may fit better. This means you have converted some of your fat tissue into lean body mass. When you stop a regular exercise program, the percentage of body fat again increases rapidly.

You may lose several pounds during an exercise session, especially in hot and humid weather. This is not fat loss. It is body water lost from sweating and must be replaced by drinking plenty of fluids. If you do not replace the water lost during exercise you can become dehydrated. This can lead to serious problems.

The most efficient way to burn fat by exercise is to: (1) exercise at an intensity that results in no shortness of breath (low intensity) and (2) exercise continuously for at least 20 to 30 minutes (long duration). This type of exercise uses stored fat as an energy source. In contrast, exercise of short duration (under 2 to 3 minutes) and high intensity (shortness of breath) uses stored carbohydrate (glycogen) as the primary energy source.

Recommended exercise for weight loss includes brisk walking, jogging, swimming, skating, cross-country skiing, cycling, jumping rope, aerobic dance or jumping on a mini-trampoline—all examples of aerobic (with oxygen) exercise. The goal is a minimum of 20 to 30 minutes of aerobic exercise 5 to 6 times a week for weight loss.

Avoid strenuous weight lifting and isometric exercise. They increase blood pressure and can be damaging to kidney and eyes and aggravate complications if you have high blood pressure or eye problems.

In summary, exercise can increase the body's sensitivity to insulin, help burn up excess calories, promote weight loss and improves blood glucose control. That is why it is important for the person with noninsulin-dependent diabetes.

How to Begin

It is important that you know how to exercise correctly and safely. Doing the right types of exercise correctly will reduce your chances of injury. Start slowly and build up endurance gradually to avoid excessive soreness.

For general fitness and blood glucose control choose activities that are aerobic. Aerobic means with oxygen, and these activities require large amounts of oxygen and involve movement of many body muscles—arms and legs. This is the type of activity that strengthens the heart and lungs, as well as burning up calories. Walking for many individuals would be an excellent type of aerobic exercise—other examples are swimming, cycling, jogging.

Anaerobic activities are the opposite of aerobic. Anaerbic means without oxygen, and you can only do them for short periods of time. Because these activities exceed the ability of the heart and lungs to deliver and process oxygen, exhaustion sets in quickly. Examples are sprinting or running up a hill or stairs.

What is an Exercise Program

An exercise program is divided into three periods: Warm-up, training (aerobic exercise) and cool-down. All are important.

Warming-up

Your warm-up period should last for about 5 to 10 minutes and prepares the body for exercise. Begin by walking in place for 30 seconds and then stetch for 5 to 10 minutes. Begin by stretching the muscles that are most often the tightest—neck, shoulders, upper and lower back—and so on down to the ankles. Stretch slowly, gently but firmly. Hold for 10 to 20 seconds and then relax. Don't bounce or stretch to the point of pain.

Aerobic Activity

This will be the main event of your exercise program, and is where you will build your endurance and overall fitness level. These improvements are known as the "training effect."

Three essential ingredients are needed to achieve a training effect:

1. Intensity refers to how hard you work during exercise. This can be determined by counting your pulse for ten seconds and multiplying by six (heart rates per minute), or by using a rating of how hard you perceive you are working. At any rate you should

always be able to talk while exercising. If you can't, you are exercising at too high a level of intensity.

To improve fitness the pulse rate must be kept within your individual target zone for at least 20 to 30 minutes of aerobic exercise. This target zone is between 70 and 85 percent of your maximal heart rate, which is the fastest your heart can beat during an all-out effort. It can be roughly estimated by subtracting your age from 220. See Table on Target Heart Rates.

2. Duration is the length of time you exercise continuously at your target heart zone. As you begin limit your workout to 10 to 15 minutes of aerobic exercise at the lower end of the target zone. Gradually increase to 20 or 30 minutes.

3. Frequency is the number of times to exercise per week. To be effective for training an exercise program must be done at least 3 to 4 times per week—spread throughout the week. For weight control exercise 5 to 6 times a week.

People with diabetes who exercise should try to do so at least every other day.

Cooling Down

Gradually decrease your heart rate by slowing down the activity. Next is the time for specific muscle strengthening exercises. This is the time to do sit-ups for strengthening stomach muscle and for push-ups to strengthen the upper body. Some people enjoy weight lifting or use of machines (e.g. Universals or Nautilus).

Complete the cool-down with more stretching exercises, similar to the ones done during warm-up. It is often helpful and enjoyable to add a relaxation period with deep breathing exercises after stretching. The cool-down should last approximately 10 to 12 minutes.

Exercise should be fun. Regular exercisers stick with it because they enjoy it. It may take time to develop this attitude toward exercises, but eventually the rewards will present themselves—"the sound of cheering from within"—and not exercising will become unthinkable.

TARGET HEART RATES

Heart Beats per ten seconds

Intensity	Age:	15	20	25	30	35	40	45	50	55	60	65	70
60%		20	20	19	19	18	18	17	17	16	16	15	15
75%		25	25	24	23	23	22	22	21	20	20	19	19
85%		29	28	27	27	26	25	25	24	23	22	22	21

Using Up Calories

Activity	120 pounds		150 pounds		220 pounds	
	Time needed to use 250 calories minutes	Calories used per hour of activity	Time needed to use 250 calories minutes	Calories used per hour of activity	Time needed to use 250 calories minutes	Calories used per hour of activity
Aerobic dancing	27	553	22	691	16	922
Badminton (singles)	47	318	38	396	28	529
Basketball	33	452	27	564	20	753
Bicycling						
6 mph	71	210	57	262	43	349
12 mhp	27	553	22	691	16	922
Bowling	100	150	83	180	71	210
Calisthenics	69	216	56	270	42	360
Canoeing (leisure)	104	144	83	180	63	240
Dancing						
Slow	89	167	71	209	54	278
Fast	27	550	22	687	16	916
Football	35	432	28	540	21	720
Golf (walking and carrying bag)	54	278	43	348	38	415
Hockey	42	360	36	420	33	450
Jumping rope	42	360	36	420	33	450
Running or jogging*						
5 mhp	34	442	27	552	20	736
7.5 mhp	24	630	19	792	14	1,050
10 mhp	18	824	15	1,030	11	1,375
Sailing	83	180	69	216	57	264
Skating (ice or roller)	61	245	49	307	37	409
Skiing						
Downhill	50	280	40	360	32	450

Activity	120 pounds		150 pounds		220 pounds	
	Time needed to use 250 calories minutes	Calories used per hour of activity	Time needed to use 250 calories minutes	Calories used per hour of activity	Time needed to use 250 calories minutes	Calories used per hour of activity
Cross-country	38	390	31	487	23	649
Soccer	45	330	37	410	29	512
Squash, racquetball	42	357	34	446	25	595
Swimming (fast freestyle)	36	420	29	522	22	698
Tennis						
Singles	42	357	34	446	25	595
Doubles	71	210	57	262	43	350
Volleyball	93	164	74	205	54	273
Walking*						
3 mph	74	206	58	258	44	344
4 mph	49	308	39	385	29	513
Upstairs	32	471	26	589	19	786
Weight training	42	340	34	420	28	520
Wrestling (practice)	23	600	18	800	14	1,020

*Walking or jogging = approximately 100 calories per mile — cover 2.5 miles for 250 calories

APPROXIMATE ENERGY EXPENDITURE
DURING PERFORMANCE OF VARIOUS ACTIVITIES
Source: Adapted from Nutrition Today,
21(2):8, 1986 with permission.

Chapter Twenty-Five
MAKE MEAL PLANNING
PART OF TRAVEL PLANNING

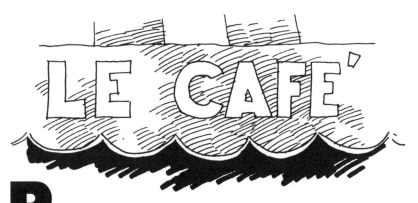

Planning is essential before taking any trip—a one day excursion, weekend camping trip or international travel. Taking appropriate precautions and planning your trip with diabetes in mind makes travel safer and more enjoyable. The following tips are offered to assist you in your planning.

Guidelines

- **Control your diabetes.** You will want to avoid insulin reactions and chances of acidosis so you can fully enjoy your time away. To do this you must do blood glucose monitoring regularly and follow your meal plan. Unfortunately, some people feel they would like to take a vacation from their diabetes when they are away from home. This could cause serious problems in a strange place.

- **Take your equipment.** Always carry insulin, syringes and appropriate blood glucose monitoring and urine ketone testing materials with you. Packing these necessities in a suitcase, however, can present tremendous problems if the suitcase is lost. Insulin does not have to be refrigerated as long as it is protected from extremes of heat or cold for prolonged periods of time. A well-supplied medical kit, containing bandages, antiseptic solution, a decongestant, motion sickness pills and sunscreen, is also invaluable to the traveler.

- **Carry identification.** Always carry a card in your wallet and wear a wristband or necklace bearing medical identification.

Travel companions should be aware that you have diabetes and should know what to do in case of an acute complication.

- **Schedules.** Schedules, whether you travel by airplane, bus, or train, are frequently upset. Delays are often encountered. Always carry extra food for these emergencies. A well planned kit with supplies for diabetes-related emergencies can prevent significant problems when traveling.

- **Changing time zones.** Prolonged airplane flights can result in considerable shifts in your diabetes management pattern. If you plan to jet across several time zones, you need advice on how to adjust your insulin.

Remember time changes occur only when you fly east or west, not north or south. Flying east, the day is shortened as you cross time zones. Flying west, the day is lengthened.

Flying east: If the day is shortened by four hours or more, and you take mixed injections of regular and intermediate-acting insulin, you may be advised to skip the intermediate-acting insulin dose that day and use regular insulin every four or five hours until the next morning when you will be back to your usual insulin dosages.

Flying west: If the day is lengthened by four hours or more you will probably be having an extra meal as well. You may then be advised to add an extra injection of regular insulin that day to cover those extra hours and meals. Again, the next day you will be back to your usual insulin dosages.

When traveling in the U.S. and the time change is only one, two, or three hours you can gradually change your morning insulin injection time. Each morning move it one-half hour ahead or behind—depending on which direction you are going—until you are back on schedule.

You may also want to consider that it may be more hazardous to become hypoglycemic when traveling than to have blood glucose which is a little less well-controlled than usual. In talking about good control, remember, it's not one or two days health professionals are talking about—it is long periods of time!

- **Immunizations.** If you travel to foreign countries that require immunizations, have the shots several weeks before departure. This will prevent you from experiencing any unfortunate side effects while you are away from home.

- **Flying.** Tell your travel agent or the airline that you have diabetes ahead of time. They can plan for a diabetic diet to be served to you as part of the in-flight service. This should be arranged several days ahead of time.

153

When boarding the plane, tell the flight attendant that you have diabetes, that you have ordered a special meal and that it's important to have your meals served on time. Have some nonperishable foods with you in your pocket, purse or flight bag—a box of raisins, dried fruit or small cans of orange or grapefruit juice are easy to carry.

- **Food and meal plans.** It is important to follow your meal plan. An exchange diet lets you substitute many different foods and still adhere to your meal plan. In this country, using exchanges is easy. However, when traveling in foreign countries you may encounter dishes that are not familiar to you. Look at ethnic cookbooks before you travel to learn about the foods used in the area you will visit. This will help you enjoy meals without difficulty. The usual concern for sanitation is as important for the person with diabetes as for the nondiabetic.

- **Translating calories.** In some foreign countries you will find "joules" listed on food labels instead of the term calories. Four joules equal one calorie.

- **Changes in meal times.** Carry food. You may not get to your destination on time. Depending on your blood glucose level, you will need approximately 10 to 15 grams of carbohydrate, which is one fruit or one starch/bread exchange, in order to delay your meal by one hour. For meals delayed more than 1½ hours, switch a later snack with the meal.

In many foreign countries, it is customary to eat late evening meals. In this case, double your afternoon snack and skip the evening snack, or have your evening snack at the usual evening meal time and your dinner late.

Another timing problem frequently occurs in Latin countries (Spain, Portugal and South America). Lunch is often served at 2 p.m. and dinner at 10 p.m. Adjust your meal plan accordingly. Have a substantial breakfast. Depending on the amount of exercise and activity planned, you may also include a late morning snack (perhaps your usual afternoon snack) between 11 a.m. and noon. Have lunch at 2 p.m., an early evening snack around 6 p.m. and then dinner at 10 p.m.

With more flexible insulin regimes available today travel and the meal time changes can be handled in an easier manner. Some insulin regimes or schedules have individuals using a longer acting insulin such as ultra lente or NPH in the evening or morning and regular insulin before meals. This type of regime may give you more flexibility with your meal times when traveling. Ask your doctor or diabetes specialist about these possibilities.

- **Changes in activities.** When traveling, you are likely to do a great deal of walking or sightseeing. You may even participate in sports. These activities require changes in your food intake and insulin if they depart from your usual activity pattern.

If you increase your activity level, it's important to include extra snacks. For moderate exercise, start with an additional fruit or starch/bread exchange for each hour of activity. For strenuous activity of long duration you may also need to decrease your insulin dose. If you have any questions contact your diabetes specialist ahead of time.

To add variety, here are some snacks you may find convenient to use while traveling. They can be used when meals are delayed, when driving or for increased activity.

Food	Quantity	Exchanges
Granola Bar	1	1 starch/bread 1 fat
Chips or snack foods	3/4 oz.	1 starch/bread 1 fat
Crackers	4 or 5 (1 oz.)	1 starch/bread 0-1 fat
Pretzels	3/4 oz.	1 starch/bread
Nuts, sunflower seeds	1 oz.	1 med. fat meat 2 fat
Dried fruit	1/4 cup (1/2 oz.)	1 fruit
Fruit rolls or bars	1	1 fruit

- **Changes in types of food.** Visit the library before you travel and check on the cuisine the country has to offer. Or check bookstores for guides to eating out in the country you will be visiting. Food is made of carbohydrates, proteins and fats wherever you travel! A leafy vegetable, even if grown in Japan instead of the U.S.A. is still one vegetable exchange. A fruit is a fruit exchange; starches or grains are starch/bread exchanges; meat, fish, cheese and eggs are still meat exchanges. And oil is a fat exchange, whether it's sesame or whale oil.

When in doubt about the portion size for a fruit or starch exchange, use 1/2 cup and you'll be safe. When in doubt about a meat exchange, use 1 oz. for 1 exchange. For a fat exchange, use 1 teaspoon. For mixed dishes such as casseroles, a 1 cup portion will be approximately 2 medium fat meat, 2 starch/bread and 1 to 2 fat exchanges. A cup of broth type soup (noodles, vegetable, rice, etc.) will be 1 starch/bread exchange and a cup of a cream based soup 1 starch/bread and 1 fat exchange. A bowl of soup

155

will be more apt to be 2 starch/breads and 1 to 2 fats for any soups.

- **Beverages can be a problem in foreign travel.** The water often is not safe to drink, and the milk may not be pasteurized. Wine in excess is not a good idea. Sugar-free soda pop may not be available, and the tea and coffee may be three-fourths cream or milk. You will probably need to use plain coffee or tea, bottled mineral water, wine in moderation and fruit juice.

- **Breakfasts are often different.** The ever popular continental breakfast usually consists of coffee, rolls and butter. If your meal plan calls for fruit and meat exchanges, supplement this with eggs, cheese, or peanut butter and fruit purchased at a local shop.

  Breakfast can be prepared in a hotel or motel room from canned fruit juice or fresh fruit, dry cereal, a bagel, bread, or a hard roll, milk and a beverage. If you plan to prepare your own meals, take along a thermos for milk.

- **Picnics can be good lunches.** For lunch you may enjoy picnicking on food purchased in grocery stores. Try meat and cheese, buns and fruit. Put them together and you have an inexpensive meal with little or no waste.

- **Food and water quality may not be consistent.** Precautions about food and water are necessary when traveling outside of the U.S. to avoid diarrhea and illness. Special care should be taken in South and Central America, Asia, Africa and Mexico.

- **Milk group**—drink boiled milk only! Avoid milk products such as ice cream and cream sauces. **Meat group**—be certain all meats are well cooked. Avoid all raw or rare meat, poultry, fish and soft cheeses. **Fruits and vegetables**—be sure to eat only the meat of fruits and vegetables. Fresh fruit should be thoroughly washed and then peeled before eating. Avoid all skins, lettuce, cabbage and other raw vegetables. Salad vegetables, which can harbor bacteria and parasites, should be thoroughly cleaned in detergent solution. Contamination can be a problem with food items displayed and sold in open markets. Poorly refrigerated foods containing mayonnaise or dairy products often harbor organisms that cause diarrhea. **Beverages**—drink purified water only and avoid ice cubes.

  Sugar-free soda pop is becoming more available the world around, but many countries still may not have it available. Many so-called "diabetic" drinks and foods in other countries are sweetened with either fructose or sorbitol. Both these sweeteners have as many calories as sugar. "Un perrier" is a sugarless mineral water with lime flavoring that may be available.

It is important to know what to do in case of illness. If illness does occur despite these precautions, see chapter 23 on meal planning during illness.

Traveler's Diarrhea. A variety of approaches are used in the prevention and treatment of traveler's diarrhea. The most important is the avoidance of food and beverages mentioned above that are likely to promote the development of diarrhea. Be sure to seek treatment at the first sign of diarrhea.

Medical Assistance for Travelers: If you should need a doctor while abroad, the International Association for Medical Assistance to Travelers (IAMAT) has set up centers in 125 countries with English- or French-speaking physicians who are on call 24 hours a day.

IAMAT publishes an annual directory of medical centers, along with the names and addresses of associated physicians who have agreed to a set payment schedule for IAMAT cardholders. For more information, write to the IAMAT membership office: 417 Center Street, Lewiston, NY 14092.

U.S. Embassies and Consultates and Time Differences. When traveling abroad U.S. consuls are also available to help you with serious medical, financial and legal difficulties. Among their many services, U.S. embassies and consulates can:

- Help you find medical assistance and inform your family and friends if you are ill or injured.

- Assist you in replacing a lost passport or visa.

- Arrange to have emergency funds sent by your family, friends, bank, or employer.

- Give you information on travel advisories, supply lists of local attorneys and notarize documents.

The following is a list of embassy addresses and phone numbers. Time differences are from Central Standard Time.

Austria:
Vienna (E), Boltzmanngasse 16; Tel (222)31-55-11
Salzburg (CG), Giselakai 51; Tel (662)28-6-01
- Time Difference: Plus 7 hours
- Emergency: 144 (first aid); 133 (police)

Belgium:
Brussels (E), 27 Blvd: du Regent; Tel (02)513-4450
- Time Difference: Plus 7 hours
- Emergency: 906 (first aid); 900 (police)

Denmark:
Copenhagen (E), Dag Hammarskjolds Alie 24; Tel (01)42 31 44
- Time Difference: Plus 7 hours
- Emergency: 000

Egypt:
Cairo (E), 5 Sharia Latin America; Tel 355-7371

Finland:
Helsinki (E), Itainen Puistotie 14A; Tel 171931
- Time Difference: Plus 8 hours
- Emergency: 000 (ambulance), 002 (police)

France:
Paris (E), 2 Avenue Gabriel; Tel 42-96-12-02
Marseille (CG), Blvd. Paul Peytral 13; Tel 91-54-92-00
Nice (CG), 31 Rue Marachel Joffre; Tel (93) 88-89-55
- Time Difference: Plus 7 hours
- Emergency: 45 67 50 50 (ambulance), 17 (police)

Germany:
Bonn (E), Deichmanns Ave.; Tel (0028) 339-3390
Berlin (M), Clayallee 170; Tel. (030) 83240 87
Frankfurt An Main (CG), Siesmayerstr. 21; Tel (0611) 740071
Munich (CG), Koeniginstr. 5; Tel (089) 23011
- Time Difference: Plus 7 hours
- Emergency: 110 (police), 55 86 61 (ambulance—Munich), 31 03 21 (ambulance—West Berlin)

Greece:
Athens (E), 91 Vasilissis Sophias Blvd.; Tel 721-2951

Ireland:
Dublin (E), 42 Elgin Road, Ballsbridge; Tel 688777

Israel:
Tel Aviv (E), 71 Hayarkon St.; Tel 03-654338
Jerusalem (CG), 18 Agron Rd.; Tel (02) 234271

Italy:
Rome (E), Via Veneto 119/A; Tel (6) 46742
Florence (CG), Lungarno Amerigo Vespucci 38; Tel (55) 298-276
Naples (CG), Piazza della Repubblica; Tel (81) 660966
- Time Difference: Plus 7 hours.
- Emergency: 7733 (ambulance) 113 (police)

Netherlands:
The Hague (E), Lange Voorhout 102; Tel (070)62-49-11
Amsterdam (CG), Museumplein 19; Tel (020) 790321
- Time Difference: Plus 7 hours
- Emergency: 555 55 55 (ambulance) 22 22 22 (police)

Norway:
Oslo (E), Drammensveien 18; Tel 44-85-50
- Time Difference: Plus 7 hours
- Emergency: 000

Portugal:
Lisbon (E), Avenida das Forcas Armadas; Tel 726-66-00

Spain:
Madrid (E), Serrano 75; Tel 276-3400
Barcelona (CG), Via Layetana 33; Tel 319-9550
- Time Difference: Plus 7 hours
- Emergency: 252 3264 (ambulance) 091 (police)

Sweden:
Stockholm (E), Strandvagen 101; Tel (08) 783-5300
- Time Difference: Plus 7 hours
- Emergency: 900 00

Switzerland:
Bern (E), Jubilaeumstr 93; Tel (031) 437011
Geneva (BO), 11, Route de Pregny; Tel (022) 990211
Zurich (CG), Zolliikerstr. 141; Tel (01) 552566
- Time Difference: Plus 7 hours
- Emergency: 144 (ambulance), 117 (police)

United Kingdom:
London, England (E), 24/31 Grosvenor Sq.; Tel (01)499-9000
Edinburgh, Scotland (CG), 3 Regent Ter.; Tel 031-556-8315
- Time Difference: Plus 6 hours
- Emergency: 999

Yugoslavia:
Belgrade (E), Kneza Milosa 50; Tel (011) 645-655

E-Embassy
CG-Consulate General
BO-Branch Office

Source: Key Officers of Foreign Service Posts; U.S. Dept. of State

Remember, your meal plan travels with you. If you follow your meal plan, anticipate travel situations and plan carefully, you can have confidence traveling.

Here are some phrases in several foreign languages that may help you when traveling.

German

I am a diabetic.	Ich bin Zuckerkrank. Ich bin Diabetiker. (M) Diabetikerin (F)
I am on a special diet.	Ich halte eine Sonderdiät ein.
I need some sugar.	Ich brauche etwas Zucker.
With sugar	Mit Zucker
Without sugar	Ohne Zucker
Sugar added	Zucker hereingestellt

Low calorie	Kalorienarm
No calories	Ohne Kalorien
Low fat	Fettarm
I take daily injections of insulin.	Täglich nehme ich Insulinspritzen
Please get me a doctor.	Rufen Sie mir bitte einen Arzt.
Sugar or orange juice, please.	Zucker oder Orangensaft, bitte.

Spanish

I am a diabetic.	Yo soy diabético (M) diabética. (F)
I am on a special diet.	Estoy a dieta especial.
I need some sugar.	Neccesito azúcar.
Without sugar	Sin azúcar
Sugar added	Con azúcar
Low calorie	Poca caloría
No calories	Sin calorías
Low fat	Poca grasa
I take daily injections of insulin.	Tomo inyecciones diarias de insulina.
Please get me a doctor.	Hágame el favor de llamar al médico.
Sugar or a glass of orange juice, please.	Azúcar o un vaso de jugo de naranja, por favor.

French

I am a diabetic.	Je suis diabétique.
I am on a special diet.	Je suis au régime spécial.
I need some sugar.	J'ai besoin de sucre.
Without sugar	Sans sucre
Sugar added	Avec le sucre
I take daily injections of insulin.	Je prends chaque jour une piqûre d'insulin.
Please get me a doctor.	Allez chercher un médecin, s'il vous plaît.
Sugar or orange juice, please.	Sucre ou jus d'orange, s'il vous plaît.

Norwegian

I am a diabetic.	Jeg har sukkersyke.
I am on a special diet.	Jeg har en spesielle diet.
I need some sugar.	Jeg trenger sukker.
With sugar	Med sukker

| Without sugar | Utenfor sukker |
| I take daily injections of insulin. | Jeg tar sproytene daglig. |

Italian

I am a diabetic.	Io sono diabetico.
Please get me a doctor.	Per favore chiama un dottore.
Sugar or orange juice, please.	Succhero o succo d'arrangio, per favore.
I take daily injections of insulin.	Predo injectiones de insulin tutti giorni.

Chapter Twenty-Six
SCHOOL LUNCH AND SNACKS—
EXCHANGE THOSE MENUS

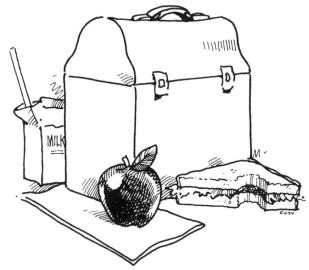

School bells signal the start of a new school year. An area of concern for students with diabetes is the lunch program. Should they carry a bag lunch or eat the school lunch?

Today many schools are becoming more nutrition conscious and are offering menus that are lower in sugar and fat. We do encourage students to use the school cafeteria whenever possible. The school lunch can serve as an example of portion control and can introduce students to a wider variety of foods. Buying school lunches also provides practice in buying and selecting food. Putting together an appropriate meal from cafeteria line options is good practice in food decision-making for the student with diabetes. There are, however, several considerations that must be kept in mind by the student who has diabetes.

It is important to check the menus ahead of time to determine if the entire menu may be used or if part of it should be replaced by foods brought from home. School lunch menus are usually published weekly in local newspapers. Encourage schools to post last minute changes in the school lunch room, so the student can be alerted to them.

To incorporate school lunch into a meal plan, the following meal plan usually works well:

2-4 starch/bread exchanges	1 fruit exchange
2 meat exchanges	1 milk exchange
0-2 vegetable exchanges	2-3 fat exchanges

This meal plan will vary with the age of the student. In the younger child (kindergarten through second grade) perhaps 2 starch/bread exchanges, 1½ meat and a smaller number of fat exchanges will be sufficient. Older students (particularly high school boys) will require additional starch/bread and perhaps milk and fat exchanges, since these are usually available for seconds. Only occasionally can students obtain more than 2 meat exchanges. Weight-watching teens may need fewer exchanges, especially fat exchanges or milk. If the food service at school is aware of the food exchanges in the student's meal plan, they are usually able to serve portions that will fulfill the student's need.

Ninety percent of the schools in the United States participate in the National School Lunch Program, which is operated by the Food and Nutrition Service of the U.S. Department of Agriculture. To qualify for federal support, schools must serve lunches that meet USDA requirements. Lunches must feature five items including the following four components.

2 oz. serving of meat or meat alternative (cheese, soy, peanut butter, vegetable protein products)

2 or more servings of vegetables or fruits or both

1 serving of whole grain or enriched bread or alternative (noodles, pasta, rice, tortillas)

1/2 pint of low fat milk

The required minimum amounts of each item served vary according to the age or grade group. Since younger children are not always able to eat the amount specified, regulations permit serving lesser amounts. For teenagers, regulations call for the serving of larger amounts of selected foods. Senior high and junior high or middle school students must choose at least three of the five food items served. Some schools are allowing grade school students to make these same choices. Some cafeteria personnel will make substitutions if they are aware a student has diabetes, for example, a fresh fruit in place of a sweet dessert.

The frequent appearance of sweet desserts in the school lunch makes following a diabetic meal plan difficult. Avoid school lunches that are high in saturated fat and sugary desserts. Occasionally, a cookie or a plain piece of cake, without icing, can be used as a starch/bread exchange. However, fresh fruit or fruit canned without the addition of sugar is usually recommended for dessert. It may need to be brought from home.

Skim milk is increasingly available in school lunches. If it isn't, the meal plan should allow for the type of milk the school serves. Currently schools must offer both low fat milk (2%) and whole milk.

In planning school lunches remember that when lunch is eaten can be as crucial as what is eaten. Secondly, lunch should be eaten at approximately the same time every day—sometime between 11:30 a.m. and 1:00 p.m. is usually best. If the school lunch is earlier the student may need two afternoon snacks—perhaps at around 2:00 or 2:30 and again around 4:00. If lunchtime is after 1:00 PM a mid-morning snack is necessary.

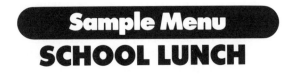

Sample Menu
SCHOOL LUNCH

The following are some examples of appropriate menus, appropriate menus with substitutions and inappropriate school lunch menus:

APPROPRIATE MENU

Food	Quantity
Pizza	2 starch/bread 2 meat
Hard roll/butter	1 starch/bread 1 fat
Tossed salad	1 vegetable
Dressing	1-2 fat
Fresh fruit	1 fruit
Low-fat milk	1 milk

Total: 3 starch/bread, 2 meat, 1 vegetable,
1 fruit, 1 milk, 2 fat exchanges

Food	Quantity
Barbecue beef on bun	1½ starch/bread 2 meat
Tater tots	1½ starch/bread 1-2 fat
Buttered carrots	1 vegetable 1 fat
Cookie	1 starch/bread
Milk	1 milk

Food	Quantity
Total: 4 starch/bread, 2 meat, 1 vegetable, 1 milk, 3-4 fat exchanges	
Need: 1 fruit exchange (or use 1 starch/bread for the fruit exchange)	

APPROPRIATE MENU WITH MODIFICATIONS

Food	Quantity
Beef ravioli	2 starch/bread 2 meat
Garlic bread	1 starch/bread 1-2 fat
Buttered green beans	1 vegetable 1 fat
Brownie	(substitute fresh fruit)
Low fat milk	1 milk

Total: 2 meat, 3 starch/bread, 1 vegetable, 1 milk, 3 fat

Need: 1 fruit exchange for substitution

INAPPROPRIATE MENU

Food	Quantity
Fried chicken	high-fat preparation
Home fries	high fat
Corn on cob/butter	OK
Peaches in heavy syrup	sugared fruit
2% chocolate milk	sugared milk

Snacks

Snacks are very important for the student with diabetes. Food must be divided into a series of meals and snacks to match the time action of insulin. Morning snacks are usually light and may consist of a fruit or starch/bread exchange or one-half pint of milk. Some students may have a small snack in the middle of the afternoon school session followed by a larger snack after arriving home. Snacks may need to be larger on days when the student has a physical education class or active recess period. Depending on the time of gym or recess snacks may be eaten before or after the activities.

Snacks may consist of fresh fruit, dried fruit, crackers, milk, a half or whole sandwich or some form of convenience food. Students should be allowed to eat as inconspicuously and with as little fuss as possible. See chapter 31 for other snack ideas.

Students with diabetes are encouraged to participate in school sports programs. This will require eating a substantial snack before practice and games. They may also need additional carbohydrates during practice or during games.

School parties frequently pose a problem for students with diabetes, because sweets should be avoided. However, **occasionally** some of these foods may be used as part of a meal plan. Here are some examples of sweets that may be counted as one starch/bread exchange plus one to two fat exchanges:

Food	Quantity
Cookie, 3″ diameter	1
Cookie, 1¾″ diameter	2
Plain cake	1 piece, 2″ square
Cupcake, without frosting	1
Angel food cake	1 small piece
Ice cream	1/2 cup
Ice milk	1/2 cup

Sugar free soda pop or Kool-Aid sweetened with artificial sweetener may be used as a free food. Dietetic hard candies can be used in limited quantities.

Other dietetic food products, such as the chocolate candies, cakes, ice cream or cookies, are not recommended. They are usually higher in calories than the foods they are replacing.

Students and parents are encouraged to educate teachers and other school personnel about diabetes. The more knowledgeable school personnel are, the more cooperative and helpful they can be.

Chapter Twenty-Seven
CHILDREN'S PARTIES

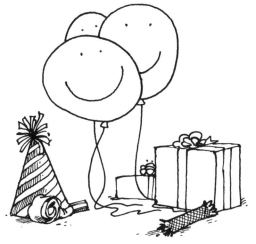

Birthday and other parties are a time of added excitement and exercise for young children. The child with diabetes may need additional food because of the increased activity. The person giving the party should know that the child has diabetes and should be told how to recognize a reaction and what to do in case of one.

Serving food before the activities and games is helpful. Then the extra food or high sugar foods can be compensated for by exercise.

For a birthday party you can use an angel food cake frosted with a low-calorie whipped topping. Sprinkle with colored sugarless beverage base (such as unsweetened Kool-Aid powder) and add candles!

Here is a workable and popular menu for a child's birthday party:

Sample Menu
CHILD'S PARTY

Hamburgers in Small Buns
(Meat and Starch/Bread Exchanges)

Carrot Sticks, Celery Sticks and Dill Pickles
(Free)

Unsweetened Fruit in Artificially Sweetened Gelatin
(Fruit Exchange)

Angel Food Cake
(Starch/Bread Exchange)

Ice Cream or Ice Milk with Waffle Cone
(Starch/Bread and Fat Exchanges) (Free)

Other Party menu ideas are:

Jell-O Eggs: Save egg shells that have been blown out. Prepare sugar-free gelatin according to package instructions. While the mixture is still liquid, pour the gelatin into egg shells. Let them set at least one day. Crack and remove the shells after gelatin has hardened. This is a free item.

Frozen Juice Cubes: Freeze fruit juice in an ice cube tray. Crush cubes in blender or food processor for fruit slush or snow cones. Four cubes equal 1 fruit exchange.

Frozen Bananas: Freeze half a banana on a stick. One of these equals 1 fruit exchange.

Sugar-Free Popsicles: See the recipe in Chapter 38.

Chapter Twenty-Eight
HOLIDAY MENUS

Sociable persons are often hosts or guests, and diabetes should not curb sociability. If a party is given at home by the person with diabetes, there should be few problems, since he or she can control the menu and the time of serving, but information about holiday and party foods can also help.

For persons taking insulin, timing of meals on holidays can be a problem. For example, if the family chooses to have the holiday meal at 2 or 3 p.m. and you are scheduled to eat at 12 noon and 6 p.m., what can you do to enjoy the holiday festivities with your family or friends? Begin by having the equivalent of your afternoon snack at 12 noon. Then at 2 or 3 p.m. have the equivalent of your lunch meal plan. Chances are that you will probably have part of your dinner meal plan at that time as well. If you do, save a portion of the evening meal plan for 6 p.m. (Doing this may throw your blood glucose tests off for that day—you may be testing closer to meal times than you normally do.)

The principle to keep in mind is this: dividing your meal plan into different sized meals and snacks won't get you into trouble as long as the total remains the same. But delay of meals will cause problems. One of the factors that determines how much insulin is needed in a day is the total number of calories eaten, and this should remain constant. Above all, remember that these changes should be reserved for very special occasions!

The same principle applies to days when you need to have your larger meal at noon instead of in the evening. For that day exchange your noon and evening meal plans.

Meal planning by the individual with diabetes depends on a

certain amount of self control as well as adequate information. With this combination, you can enjoy a normal social life and even "have a ball!"

These menu suggestions may help your holiday planning. Recipes for the starred items are found in Chapter 38. The number of exchanges you count in your meal plan will depend upon the amount you decide to eat.

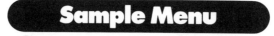

THANKSGIVING

Tomato-Beef Bouillon
(1/2 tomato juice and 1/2 beef bouillon)
with Dill Weed and Sliced Lemon
(Free)

Roast Turkey	Dressing
(Meat Exchange)	(Starch/Bread and Fat Exchange)
Gravy	Mashed Potatoes
(Fat Exchange)	(Starch/Bread Exchange)

Cauliflower Supreme*
(Vegetable, Fruit and Fat Exchanges)

Cranberry-Celery Salad*
(Free)

Rolls	Margarine
(Starch/Bread Exchange)	(Fat Exchange)

Pumpkin Pie* with Low Calorie Whipped Topping
(Milk, Vegetable and Fat Exchanges)

Coffee	Milk
(Free)	(Milk Exchange)

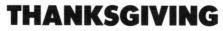

CHRISTMAS

Hors d'oeuvres:

Sparkling Punch
(Artificially Sweetened Cranberry Cocktail and
Fresca — 1/2 and 1/2)
(Free)

Fresh Vegetable Slices
(Free)

with

Cottage Cheese Dip
(Cottage cheese pureed in blender with
onions, parsley and seasonings)
(Meat Exchange)

Dinner:

Roast Beef Au Jus
(Meat Exchange)

Browned Potatoes   String Beans with Mushrooms
(Starch/Bread and Fat Exchanges)   (Vegetable Exchange)

Garden Green Salad with Low Calorie Dressing
(Free)

Rolls   Margarine
(Starch/Bread Exchange)   (Fat Exchange)

Flaming Cherries Jubilee*
(Fruit, Starch/Bread and Fat Exchanges)

Coffee   Milk
(Free)   (Milk Exchange)

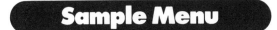

Sample Menu

EASTER

Baked Ham
(Baste with sugar-free ginger ale)
(Meat Exchange)

Escalloped Potatoes   Fresh Asparagus Spears
(Starch/Bread and Fat Exchanges)   (Vegetable Exchange)

Carrot Orange Toss*
(Fruit and Vegetable Exchanges)

Rolls   Margarine
(Starch/Bread Exchange)   (Fat Exchange)

Fresh Strawberry Shortcake
with
Low Calorie Whipped Topping
(Fruit and Starch/Bread Exchanges)

Coffee   Milk
(Free)   (Milk Exchange)

171

4th OF JULY

Backyard Barbecue

Chicken on the Grill
(Meat Exchange)

Potato Salad
(Starch/Bread and Fat Exchanges)

Grilled Vegetable Kabobs
(Cherry Tomatoes, Zucchini, Mushroom, Small Onion)

Relishes
(Vegetable Exchange)

Rolls
(Starch/Bread Exchange)

Margarine
(Fat Exchange)

Marshmallow Crispies*
(Fruit Exchange)

Watermelon
(Fruit Exchange)

Low Calorie Lemonade
(Free)

Sugar-Free Pop
(Free)

Part IV

GUIDELINES FOR FOOD PURCHASING AND PREPARATION

Chapter Twenty-Nine
FOOD LABELS CAN BE BOTH HELPFUL AND MISLEADING

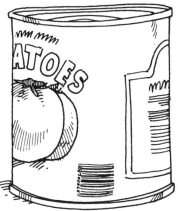

Labels can help you decide which foods are appropriate to use in meal planning and how to use them correctly. Regulations regarding food labels that can be helpful are: ingredients must be listed in descending order according to the percentage of weight they contribute to the total product; if a manufacturer makes a nutrition claim or adds nutrients to a food, a complete nutrition label must be added; misleading photographs are unlawful; a few terms such as "low sodium" or "low calorie" are specifically defined by federal regulation.

There still is, however, a considerable amount of information that is not given to us. Many of the almost 3,000 additives in current use do not need to be specifically named. A so-called "natural food" can still contain artificial ingredients. Foods "with no salt" can still have sodium. Furthermore, most consumers aren't aware that the term "light" may refer to a product's color or density rather than its calorie or fat content! Many "sugar-free" products have as many or more calories as their sugared counterparts. Label reading is further complicated by the fact that only slightly more than one-half the food products on supermarket shelves have any nutrition labeling at all.

The food labeling of food products other than meat and poultry is regulated by the Food and Drug Administration (FDA). The U.S. Department of Agriculture (USDA) regulates meat and poultry products.

Three general guidelines can help you make decisions about which foods to purchase:

1. Look closely at the descriptive terms used on the label (i.e., low calorie, low sodium, light, etc.). Some can be helpful, some can be misleading.
2. Look at the list of ingredients. They will tell you what is contained in a product and will help you decide whether you should use a particular product.
3. Look for nutritional labeling. This information can help you fit the product into your meal plan.

Your First Clue: Food Labeling Terms

Recent changes in regulations for food labeling terms have helped consumers be sure they are getting what they think they are buying. However, there are still terms that are ambiguous, and some are downright misleading. Some clues are still hard to decipher!

Some food labeling terms are well regulated and clearly specify how the term can be used. Other food labeling terms can be confusing or misleading to the consumer. First, let's look at terms regulated by the FDA.

"Low calorie": These foods may contain no more than 40 calories per serving or no more than 0.4 calorie per gram. (Serving size can vary, however.) Foods naturally low in calories (such as vegetables) cannot be called "low calorie." They can be labeled "vegetables, a low-calorie food."

"Reduced calorie": These foods must have one-third fewer calories than the standard product and must include a comparison of the standard and reduced-calorie version on the labels.

"Diet" or "dietetic": These foods must meet the same requirements as "low calorie" or "reduced calorie" foods and must contain no more than 40 calories per serving or have at least one-third fewer calories than the regular product. However, they can be low in sodium only, not calories. In that case they will still be labeled "diet" but do not need to meet the requirements of "low calorie" or "reduced calorie" foods.

"Sodium-free": These foods must have less than 5 mg. of sodium per serving.

"Very-low sodium": Foods that have no more than 35 mg. of sodium per serving.

"Low sodium": Foods that contain no more than 140 mg. of sodium per serving.

"Reduced sodium": Sodium levels that have been reduced by at least 75 percent. The level must show the "before" and "after" sodium levels.

"Enriched" or "fortified": Products that contain added vitamins, minerals, or protein. The labels must have full nutritional disclosure; "per serving" amounts of nutrients must be given.

"Imitation": The product is nutritionally inferior—that is, lower in protein, vitamins, or minerals. Foods that are lower in calories, fat, or cholesterol are not considered imitation.

The USDA regulates meat, poultry and egg products. Fat claims, such as "lite," "lean," and "extra lean" have been used interchangeably on meat and poultry products containing 25 percent less fat than a comparable product and on products containing no more than 10 percent fat. Under the new policy the following terms are specified:

"Extra lean": These foods contain less than 5 percent fat.

"Lean" and "low fat": Contain less than 10 percent fat.

"Lite," "Leaner," and "Lower fat": Contain at least 25 percent less fat than similar products.

The following terms are either not regulated or if they are regulated they can be misleading to you as you read labels.

"Light" or "lite": These terms, when applied to food products other than meat or poultry, can mean anything from a lighter color or texture to less sodium, calories, or fat.

"Sugar-free" or "sugarless": Although these foods cannot contain sucrose (table sugar) they can have other sweeteners, including honey, corn syrup, fructose, sorbitol, or mannitol. If these foods aren't low in calories, the label must state that it is not a reduced-calorie food. Be wary of ice cream, candy bars, and cakes that are labeled "sugar-free" or "sugarless." These products are usually equal or even higher in calories than the products they are replacing. They are often sweetened with sorbitol, which is the alcohol form of glucose. It contains four calories per gram, just as does other carbohydrate. Because sorbitol is not soluble in water, the fat content of these products is usually increased in order to dissolve the sorbitol. Products containing sorbitol can also cause diarrhea.

"Low salt": Since salt is not the only ingredient that contains sodium, a food that is low in salt is not necessarily low in sodium. Terms such as unsalted, salt-free, no salt, no salt added, without added salt, or no salt added during processing all refer to salt, but the food could have significant levels of sodium either naturally or from substances added for preservation, leavening, or other purposes.

"No cholesterol": These are food products that do not contain cholesterol. Remember, however, only foods from animal sources contain cholesterol. Vegetable sources never do. Cholesterol-free foods are not necessarily low in fat or saturated fat.

"Natural": No guarantee unless it is a meat or poultry product. The FDA does not have regulations on the word "natural."

"Organic": This term also has no legal meaning. It can be used without any guides.

Your Second Clue: Ingredient Listing

Ingredients in a product are listed on the label in descending order of predominance by weight. The ingredient contained in the largest amount is listed first and so on down the list. If sugar is the first, possibly the second ingredient on the label, the product contains a large amount of sugar and probably should be avoided. If sugar is the fourth, fifth, or sixth ingredient, there is usually such a small amount that it doesn't matter.

Some ingredients are of concern because they are similar to sugar. Words ending in "ose" are generally forms of sugar. Sugar used in cooking and at the table is sucrose; other sugars are dextrose, fructose, levulose, lactose and glucose. Check to see how many of these ingredients are in the product, because all are forms of sugar. See chapters 32 and 33 for more information about sugars and alternative sweeteners.

Adding water may reduce the percentage of sugar without actually changing the amount in the product. Percentages can be misleading. As an example, a glass of cola has a lower percentage of sugar than a bouillon cube but actually contains significantly more sugar. It is more helpful to know the actual number of grams of sugar contained in the product.

Another phrase used on the ingredient list is "nutritive sweetener." This identifies a sweetener containing calories. Examples of nutritive sweeteners are: invert sugar, corn syrup, corn sugar, dextrin, molasses, sorghum, honey, maple or brown sugar.

If the list contains the phrase "non-nutritive sweetener," it indicates the sweetener contains few or no calories. Examples are saccharin and aspartame (trade names Equal® or NutraSweet®).

Besides sugar you should be aware of ingredients that are high in saturated fat. Some of these are: animal, bacon, beef, or chicken fat; butter; cocoa butter or chocolate; coconut or coconut oil; hardened or hydrogenated shortenings, fats, or oil; lard; and palm or palm kernel oil.

If you have been advised to limit your sodium intake be on the lookout for the following high sodium ingredients: bouillon, brine (salt and water), broth, monosodium glutamate, salt, soy sauce.

In summary, check the ingredient list for the order of ingredients and ingredients you want to limit or avoid.

Third Clue: Nutritional Labeling

Next look for nutritional labeling. This information can help you fit the product into your meal plan. Nutritional labeling is voluntary for most products. However, it is required for any food product for which special nutritive claims are made or to which extra nutrients are added.

Any company that offers nutritional labeling must follow a standard format. The label must state the serving size and the number of servings per container. It also must state calories, grams of carbohydrate, protein, fat, milligrams of sodium, and percentages of important vitamins and minerals per serving. Other information such as milligrams of cholesterol, grams of saturated and polyunsaturated fat is optional.

The following are examples of nutritional labeling:

ENRICHED HARD ROLLS
Nutrition Information
(per serving)
Serving = 1 roll
Servings per container = 6

Calories...............160
Protein ....5 gms.
Carbohydrate......30 gms.
Fat.................2 gms.
Sodium ....155 mg.

**Percentage of U.S. Recommended
Daily Allowances (U.S. RDA)**

Protein	8	Niacin	8
Vitamin A	0	Calcium	2
Vitamin C	0	Iron	6
Thiamine (B$_{12}$)	10		
Riboflavin (B$_6$)	6		

DRY ROASTED PEANUTS
Nutrition Information
(per serving)
Serving size = 1 ounce
Servings per container = 8

Calories 160
Protein ....7 gms.
Carbohydrate ....6 gms.
Fat (71% of calories)
   from fat............14 gms.
   Polyunsaturated ....5 gms.
   Saturated ....2 gms.
Cholesterol ....0 mg.
Sodium ....250 mg.

Percentage of U.S. Recommended Daily Allowances (U.S. RDA)

Protein 10	Niacin 10
Vitamin A 0	Calcium 0
Vitamin C 0	Iron 2
Thiamine (B_{12}) 0	
Riboflavin (B_6) 2	

Knowing the number of calories per serving can be helpful in deciding how to fit a product into your meal plan. If a food contains less than 20 calories per serving, it may be used as a free food either at mealtime or snacktime. However, free foods, if they contain calories, should be limited to one per meal or not more than three per day.

Products that might be useful are artificial sweeteners, diet pops, dietetic gelatins and puddings, and fruits canned without added sugar. Products that may be useful as free foods include diet syrups, diet jams or jellies, diet hard candies and sugar-free gum.

Using Nutritional Labeling

In order to use the information from nutritional labeling effectively, you must first understand the basis for grouping foods into exchange lists. The indicated amount of each food in a single group contains approximately the same number of calories and grams of carbohydrate, protein, and fat. By looking at the nutrition information on the label, you can estimate how many exchanges are in a serving of a food and how to include it in your meal plan. You must pay particular attention to the grams of carbohydrate, protein, and fat, but the grams do not need to be exactly equal. Variations of a few calories or grams of protein, carbohydrate, or fat are usually not significant.

The following table may be used to convert the information on a label to the exchange system.

Exchange	Calories	Carbo-hydrate	Protein	Fat
1 starch/bread	80	15 gms.	3 gms.	trace
1 lean meat	55	—	7 gms.	3 gms.
1 medium-fat meat	75	—	7 gms.	5 gms.
1 high-fat meat	100	—	7 gms.	8 gms.
1 vegetable	25	5 gms.	2 gms.	—
1 fruit	60	15 gms.	—	—
1 milk (skim)	90	12 gms.	8 gms.	trace
1 fat	45	—	—	5 gms.

Steps to Convert Nutritional Labeling to Exchanges

The following label is from a 10 oz. box of frozen pizza

Nutrition information per serving

Serving size............................	1/2 pizza (5 oz.)
Servings per container...................	2
Calories	350
Protein.................................	18 gms.
Carbohydrate...........................	33 gms.
Fat	16 gms.

To convert label information to the exchange system, follow these steps:

1. Check the label for the information you need to convert to the exchange system. You need:

serving size—1/2 pizza
calories—350
carbohydrate—33 grams
protein—18 grams
fat—16 grams

2. Check for serving size. Is this a reasonable size for your use?

3. Compare the label information with the carbohydrate, protein, fat and calories on the exchange table. First, convert the grams of carbohydrate in your serving size to exchanges. In this case, 33 grams of carbohydrate would be 2 starch/bread exchanges.

	Carbohydrate	Protein	Fat
1/2 pizza	33 gms.	18 gms.	16 gms.
2 starch/bread	30 gms.	6 gms.	—

4. Next, subtract the grams of protein you used in converting the carbohydrate to exchanges. Then convert the grams of protein you have remaining to meat exchanges. Use the medium-fat meat exchange values.

	Carbohydrate	Protein	Fat
1/2 pizza	33 gms.	18 gms.	16 gms.
2 starch/bread	30 gms.	-6 gms.	—
		12 gms.	16 gms.
2 med. fat meat exchanges		14 gms.	10 gms.

5. Next, subtract the grams of fat in the meat exchanges from the fat contained in the serving size. Then convert the remaining grams of fat to fat exchanges.

	Carbohydrate	Protein	Fat
1/2 pizza	33 gms.	18 gms.	16 gms.
2 starch/bread	30 gms.	-6 gms.	—
		12 gms.	16 gms.
2 med. fat meat exchanges		14 gms.	-10 gms.
			6 gms.
1 fat exchange			5 gms.

6. If you eat 1/2 of this 10 oz. pizza, you use the following exchanges from your meal plan:

> 2 starch/bread, 2 medium-fat meat, 1 fat

7. Final check:

	Carbohydrate	Protein	Fat	Calories
1/2 pizza	33 gms.	18 gms.	16 gms.	350
Exchanges: 2 starch/bread 2 med. fat meat 1 fat	30 gms.	20 gms.	15 gms.	355

8. If the difference between the grams per serving and the grams accounted for by the exchanges system is less than one-half of an exchange, you do not need to count those extra grams.

Marketing Tricks

In the competitive food industry where for every man, woman, and child there is almost $1,300 worth of food to choose from, manufacturers will try all kinds of subtle, and some not so subtle, tactics to encourage consumers to buy their products. Many package labels are little more than advertisements for food manufacturers rather than straightforward information from which consumers can make choices based on the nutritional quality of products.

Food labeling has come a long way since the first legislation against deceptive labeling was introduced 30 years ago. Nutritional labeling was a big step forward. However, it is still important to not reach for a package that looks healthful because of its coloring, lettering style or bold claims.

Chapter Thirty
FITTING CONVENIENCE INTO YOUR MEAL PLAN

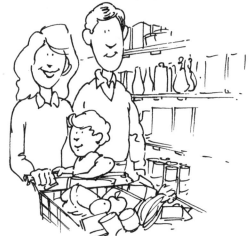

In our busy society, convenience can be one of the main influences on the way we order our lives, and particularly on our eating habits. If we're not grabbing a bite at a fast-food restaurant, we're looking for a meal that is quick and easy to prepare so that we can spend as much time as possible on other pursuits.

Convenience foods are the fastest growing processed food group today, because they give us what we demand: quick, easy-to-prepare, good-tasting, and relatively inexpensive meals.

But aside from convenience, there are other things that we consumers care a great deal about. We are becoming more knowledgeable about nutrition and the effects that different foods have on our health. We want to eat not only for energy to enjoy our daily activities, but also to ensure our health throughout a long and productive life. Unfortunately, the goals of convenience and good nutrition are not always easily achieved together. The following guidelines can help you meet your nutritional goals while enjoying the convenience of convenience foods!

Goal: Limiting calories to reduce weight.

A weight control program that is low in calories as well as nutritionally adequate should provide 1200-1500 calories a day. Of these calories, about 400 to 500 calories, or a third of the total, should be consumed at dinner. For weight maintenance, many adults' meal plans will be based on an intake of approximately 1800 to 2400 calories, or approximately 600 to 800 calories at dinner. Look at the nutritional label or **Convenience Food Facts** to see how many calories are in the food product.

Goal: Reduce fat content of diet.

Use foods that have the number of fat exchanges allowed in your meal plan. (Five grams of fat is equal to a teaspoon of fat or one fat exchange.) Foods high in fat ae also high in total calories. If 30% of your calories are from fat, the total fat content of the meal on a weight control diet will be between 15 and 18 grams of fat; on a weight maintenance diet, it will be 20 to 28 grams of fat. Please remember that you can move fat exchanges from one meal or snack to another. If you know you will need more fat exchanges at dinner go easy on your fat exchanges earlier in the day.

Goal: Reducing salt content of diet.

Many convenience foods are high in salt content. Salt is usally added not to preserve the food, but to satisfy the public's desire for a salty taste. It has been recommended that Americans limit their daily sodium intake to approximately 1,000 to 3,000 milligrams. Per meal, sodium should not exceed 1,000 milligrams; people on sodium-restricted diets should consume less than 700 milligrams per meal.

Goal: Maintain your meal plan.

The following chart gives you average exchange values for several popular convenience foods. For complete information on convenience foods, their calorie and carbohydrate, protein, and fat amounts see **Convenience Food Facts,** in which Arlene Monk, R.D., has listed many popular convenience foods for you.

Expanded Food List
CONVENIENCE FOODS

Exchange Values for Favorite Convenience Foods

Product	Serving Size	Exchanges
Frozen Dinners:		
Chicken Chow Mein	11 oz.	3 starch/bread 1 lean meat
Fried Chicken	11 oz.	3½ starch/bread 1½ med. fat meat 1 vegetable 3 fat

Exchange Values for Favorite Convenience Foods

Product	Serving Size	Exchanges
Lite Dinners	8-11 oz.	2 starch/bread 2 lean meat 1 vegetable
Turkey	11 oz.	2 starch/bread 2 lean meat 1 vegetable
Entrees:		
Frozen burritos	1	2 starch/bread 1/2 med. fat meat 1 fat
Chili	1 cup (8 oz.)	2 starch/bread 2 med. fat meat 1/2 fat
Breaded fish fillets or sticks	1 fillet or 3 sticks (3 oz.)	1 starch/bread 1 med. fat meat 2-3 fat
Hamburger Helper	1 serving	2 starch/bread 2 med. fat meat 1 fat
Macaroni and cheese	1 cup (8 oz.)	2 starch/bread 1 med. fat meat 1 fat
Meat pies	8 oz.	3 starch/bread 1 med. fat meat 3 fat
Frozen pizza	1/4 of 23 oz. pizza	2 starch/bread 1½ med. fat meat 2 fat
Light Seafood Entrees, frozen	9-10 oz.	1 starch/bread 2 lean meat 1 vegetable
Spaghetti and Meatballs	1 cup (8 oz.)	2 starch/bread 1 med. fat meat 1 fat
Accompaniments:		
Noodles or rice and sauce (as prepared)	1½ cup	1½-2 starch/bread 1 fat
Pasta Salad, as prepared (Suddenly Salads)	1/6 pkg.	1 starch/bread 1 fat
Au gratin potatoes	1/2 cup	1½ starch/bread 1 fat

Exchange Values for Favorite Convenience Foods

Product	Serving Size	Exchanges
Stuffing mixes	1/2 cup	1½ starch/bread 1-2 fat
Breads:		
Dinner rolls	1	1 starch/bread 1/2 fat
Quick bread mixes	1/16 loaf	1 starch/bread 1 fat
Muffins	1 small	1 starch/bread 1 fat
	1 medium	2 starch/bread 1-2 fat
Soups:		
Chunky soups	1 can (10¾ oz.)	1 starch/bread 1 vegetable 1 med. fat meat
Regular soups	1 cup	1 starch/bread (plus 1 fat for cream soups)
Snacks:		
Corn chips	1 oz.	1 starch/bread 2 fat
Snack crackers	8 (1 oz.)	1 starch/bread 1-2 fat
Fruit roll-ups	1 roll (1/2 oz.)	1 fruit
Granola bar	1 bar	1 starch/bread 1 fat
Nuts and sunflower seeds	1 oz.	1 med. fat meat 2 fat
Microwave popcorn	2 cups, popped	1 starch/bread 2 fat
Lite syrup	1 oz.	1 fruit
Beverages:		
Hot cocoa mixes (sugar free)	1 pkg.	1 starch/bread **or** 1 skim milk

Chapter Thirty-One
SMART SNACKING

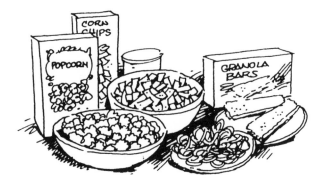

Although snacking often has a "bad name," snacks can be very helpful in the regulation of blood glucose levels. Snacks can provide an additional source of carbohydrates, protein, and fat for your body. Often these energy producing nutrients consumed at one meal may not cover your body's energy needs until the next meal. Without a snack your blood glucose can easily drop too low, causing hypoglycemia.

If you use insulin, carefully timed and appropriate snacks can be especially important. You need to work them into your meal plan to counteract the effect of insulin peaking. For example, a morning injection of intermediate-acting insulin may be at its greatest level of activity at 3 to 4 in the afternoon. Eating a snack at that time boosts your blood glucose and reduces the chance of an insulin reaction.

The need to snack depends on your insulin regime, age, activity level, calorie needs, etc. In general, young children and active people using insulin do well with a mid-morning, mid-afternoon and bedtime snack. Some kids even do better with two afternoon snacks, depending on their school lunch and their dinner times.

Most people who use insulin need an afternoon and evening snack to cover their energy needs over these longer spans of time.

In addition to knowing when to snack, you also need to know what and how much to eat. Eating too much or an inappropriate snack can cause blood sugars to soar and also contribute significant calories that you may not need!

Planning for Snacks

Many commercial snacks are made with animal fats or hydrogenated vegetable fats and are high in sodium. They contribute a significant amount of fat, salt and calories to the diets of many people. Sale of salty snacks is a $6.1 billion dollar industry. The average American household consumes 28.6 pounds of salty snacks per year. Of this amount, 44.1% is potato chips, 24.1% corn tortilla chips, 14.9% salted nuts, 5.2% salted meat snacks, 4.8% pretzels, 4.6% other salted snacks, and 2.3% popcorn.

The following are hints for choosing snack foods:

- Choose your foods carefully. Avoid empty calorie snacks that are high in sugar, fat, salt, and calories, but low in nutrients.

- Buy or prepare snacks that are low in sodium and fat. If high sodium and fatty snacks are not in the house they will be hard to eat.

- When you have time to prepare your own snacks, modify your recipes. Cut down the amount of sugar and use skim milk, margarine, oils, egg whites or egg substitutes.

- When preparing other snacks, try seasoning with spices such as basil, dill, lemon juice and garlic or onion powder instead of salt. Use fruit juices as a sweetener.

- If you are trying to lose weight, avoid nuts, seeds, dried fruits and modified sweets that may be healthful but not necessarily helpful in reducing calories.

- Snack on foods that contain complex carbohydrate and fiber. They contribute nutrients, such as vitamins and minerals as well as calories. Keep fruits and vegetables on hand in the refrigerator. They make excellent snacks.

- Beware of commercially manufactured snack foods, energy bars, etc. They are frequently similar to candy bars and often are scarcely more than fat, sugar and salt with a little flavoring.

- Examine the ingredient list and nutrition labeling on purchased snack items.

- Plan ahead to make sure you have appropriate and appealing snacks available.

- If your meal plan includes snacks, don't skip them.

The following are ideas for some healthy snack choices. For more ideas see **The Joy of Snacks** by Nancy E. Cooper, R.D..

Alternative Snack Choices:

Bread or toast (whole grain), bagels, English muffins, breadsticks

Cereal snack mix (prepare with margarine, garlic powder and
    Worcestershire sauce)

Cookies (homemade using whole grains, oils and minimal sugar)

Crackers

> No-fat commercial choices: Finn Crisps, flatbread, hardtack,
>   Matzo, Wasa Brod, Akmak

> Low fat commercial choices: bread sticks, melba toast, Ry
>   Krisps, zwieback, graham crackers, oyster crackers, saltines,
>   soda crackers

Dried fruits: apricots, dates, prunes, raisins

Frozen yogurt

Fruits and real fruit juices (fresh, frozen or canned in fruit juice)

Fruit and nut breads (prepared with whole grains, oils, and minimal
    sugar)

Fruit roll-ups, fruit bars and fruit jerky

Low fat commercial snacks: animal crackers, gingersnaps, fig bars,
    graham crackers, molasses cookies.

Nuts (unsalted and roasted)

Peanut butter

Peanuts (unsalted and roasted)

Popcorn (air-popped or popped in acceptable vegetable oils, served
    plain, lightly salted or sprinkled with Parmesan cheese)

Pretzels (unsalted)

Sandwiches

Seeds (unsalted and roasted)

Soybeans (unsalted and roasted)

Trail mix (unsalted popcorn, raisins, unsalted peanuts, dates and
    dried fruits such as apricots, peaches, pears, and pineapple)

Vegetables (raw, cooked or served with low fat dips)

    Sometimes what is healthy and best just isn't convenient! For
those occasions the following "Legal Junk Foods" may help you
make the best choice available. It is always important to weigh
convenience and necessity against the ideal—there are times when
you will go with convenience. This list is for those occasions!

"Legal Junk Foods!"

Food	Serving Size	Exchanges
Starch/Bread		
Animal crackers	8	1 starch/bread
Bread sticks		
8" long, 1/2" diam.	2	1 starch/bread
4" long, 1/4" diam.	6	1 starch/bread
Cheetos, Corn Chips	3/4 oz.	1 starch/bread 2 fat
Fritos, Doritos, Cheese Nips	20	1 starch/bread 1 fat
Cheez-Its	27	1 starch/bread 1 fat
Snack Cracker Mixes	1 oz. or 1/3 cup	1 starch/bread 1 fat
Fruit Sorbet	1/2 cup	2 starch/bread **or** 2 fruit
Fruit Ice	1/2 cup	2 starch/bread **or** 2 fruit
Muffin, plain, blueberry, or bran (as prepared from mix, 1/12 mix)	1	1 starch/bread 1 fat
Popcorn, no fat added	3 cups popped	1 starch/bread
Microwave popcorn	2 cups	1 starch/bread 2 fat
Potato chips	15 or 3/4 oz.	1 starch/bread 2 fat
Pretzels, very thin sticks	(3/4 oz.) 67	1 starch/bread
very thin twisted, (3-ring)	(3/4 oz.) 4	1 starch/bread
Raisin, nut, coconut fruit mix (trail mixes)	1 oz. or 1/4 cup	1 starch/bread 1 fat
Rice cakes	2 cakes	1 starch/bread
Ritz, Hi Ho crackers, etc.	7	1 starch/bread 1 fat
Pepperidge Farm Goldfish Crackers	25 or 1/2 oz.	1/2 starch/bread 1/2 fat
Ry Krisp	3 triple crackers	1 starch/bread
Cup of Soup (broth type)	1 package	1/2 starch/bread
Cup of Soup (cream type)	1 package	1/2 starch/bread 1/2 fat

Food	Serving Size	Exchanges
Triscuit Wafers or other snack crackers	6 to 8 (1 oz.)	1 starch/bread 1-2 fat
Wheat Snacks	10 crackers	1 starch/bread 1 fat
Wheat Thins	16	1 starch/bread 1 fat
Whole Wheat crackers, no fat added (such as Finn, Kavli, Wasa)	2-4 slices (3/4 oz.)	1 starch/bread
*Ginger Snaps	3	1 starch/bread
*Lorna Doone Shortbread	3	1 starch/bread
*Vanilla Wafers	6	1 starch/bread 1 fat
*Frozen yogurt	1/3 cup	1 starch/bread
*Granola bar (not dipped or coated)	1 small	1 starch/bread 1 fat
*Pudding pop	1	1 starch/bread 1/2 fat
*Family Style Cookies	1	1 starch/bread
Meat		
Beef Jerky	1/2 oz.	1 lean meat
Cheese Spread	1 oz.	1 med. fat meat
Breaded Mozzarella Cheese Nuggets	3 oz.	1 starch/bread 2 med. fat 1 fat
String Cheese	1 oz.	1 med. fat meat
Chicken Dipsters	3 oz.	1 starch/bread 2 med. fat meat 1 fat
*Nuts or seeds (peanuts, sunflower seeds, etc.)	1/4 cup or 1 oz.	1 med. fat meat 2 fat
Snack Mate	1 oz.	1 med. fat meat
Fruit		
Apple cider, unsweetened	1/2 cup	1 fruit
Catawba juice	1/2 cup	1 fruit
Cranapple juice, low-calorie	1½ cups	1 fruit
Hawaiian Punch, low-calorie	1½ cups	1 fruit
Fruit bars	1	1½ fruit
Fruit and cream bars	1 bar	1½ fruit
Fruit n' juice bars	1 bar	1 fruit

Food	Serving Size	Exchanges
Fun Fruits, Real Fruit Snacks	1 pouch	1½ fruit
Fruit roll-ups or rolls	1 (1/2 oz.)	1 fruit
Fruit Snacks, Sierra Trail Mix	1 pouch, .9 oz.	1 starch/bread 1 fat
Fruit Snacks, Tropical	1 pouch, .9 oz.	1½ fruit
Fruit Jerky	1	1 fruit
Dried Fruit	1/2 oz. or 1/4 cup	1 fruit
Gelatin Pops	1	1/2 fruit
Raisins	1/2 oz. or 1 small box	1 fruit
Tomato juice	1 cup	1 fruit
Weight Watchers Apple Snacks or Fruit Snacks	1 package (1/2 oz.)	1 fruit
Milk		
Alba 66 or Alba 77	1 envelope	1 starch/bread **or** 1 skim milk
Hot Cocoa Mix, sugar-free	1 envelope	1 starch/bread **or** 1 skim milk
*Chocolate Skim Milk	1 cup	1 starch/bread 1 skim milk 1/2 fat
Instant Breakfast, sugar-free	1 envelope	1 skim milk (mixed with 8 oz. skim milk = 2 skim milk)
Puddings made with skim milk, reduced calorie or sugar free	1/2 cup	1 starch/bread 1 skim milk
Weight Watcher's Yogurt	1 cup	1 fruit 1 skim milk

*Recommended for occasional use only due to high sugar and/or fat content.

Chapter Thirty-Two
SUGAR DISGUISES

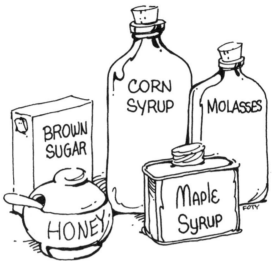

Here is a brief explanation of the more common sugars and sweeteners. Read labels carefully and note where on the ingredient list these products are listed. If they are first, possibly second, or if there are many of these different terms on the label, sugar is present in a large amount. It may be best to avoid the product. If at the end of the ingredient listing, don't worry about it.

Brown Sugar: Consists of sugar crystals contained in a molasses syrup with natural flavor and color, or it may be made by simply adding syrup to refined white sugar in a mixture. It has 91 to 96 percent sucrose.

Corn Syrup: Produced by the action of enzymes and/or acids on cornstarch. It is the liquid form of corn sugar and, when crystallized, may be called corn syrup solids or corn sweetener. High fructose corn syrup is a derivative of corn. The amounts of fructose vary with the manufacturer; these syrups may contain 42, 55 or 90 percent fructose. Dextrose comprises most of the balance.

Dextrin: A sugar formed by the partial breakdown of starch.

Dextrose: Also called corn sugar. It is made commercially from starch by the action of heat and acids, or enzymes. It is often sold blended with regular sugar.

Fructose: Also called fruit sugar or levulose. It occurs naturally in small quantities in fruit. It has four calories per gram, as do all carbohydrates.

Galactose: Simple sugar found in lactose (milk sugar).

Glucose: The basic simple sugar found in the blood, which is either absorbed in this digested form or manufactured in the body from other sources. It is the form of carbohydrate that the body uses for energy.

Honey: An invert sugar formed by an enzyme from nectar gathered by bees. Its composition and flavor depend on the source of nectar. Fructose, glucose, maltose and sucrose are among its components.

Invert Sugar: A sugar formed by splitting sucrose into its component parts: glucose and fructose. This is done by an application of acids or enzymes. It is used only in liquid form and is sweeter than sucrose. Invert sugar helps prolong the freshness of baked foods and confections and is useful in preventing food shrinkage.

Lactose: The sugar found in milk, which is a combination of glucose and galactose. It is made from whey and skim milk for commercial purposes. The pharmaceutical industry is a primary user of prepared lactoses.

Maltose: Comes from the breakdown of starch in the malting of barley.

Mannitol: A sugar alcohol manufactured from mannose and galactose. It is half as sweet as sucrose.

Mannose: Comes from manna and the ivory nut, used mainly by sugar chemists.

Maple Syrup: A syrup made by concentrating the sap of the sugar maple tree.

Molasses: The thick, brown syrup that is separated from raw sugar in its manufacture.

Raw Sugar: Tan to brown in appearance, it is a course, granulated solid obtained by evaporating the moisture from sugar cane juice.

Sorbitol: A sugar alcohol made commercially from glucose or dextrose, about half as sweet as sucrose.

Sorghum: Syrup from the sweet juice of the sorghum grain.

Sucrose: Crystals from cane or beet sugars. It is composed of two simple sugars, glucose and fructose. Sucrose is about 99.9 percent pure and sold either granulated, cubed or powdered.

Turbinado Sugar: Sometimes viewed erroneously as raw sugar. It actually has to go through a refining process to remove impuritiess and most of the molasses. It is produced by separating raw sugar crystals and washing them with steam.

Xylitol: A sugar alcohol manufactured from xylose (wood sugar from part of the birch tree). Its sweetness is about equal to sucrose.

Chapter Thirty-Three
ALTERNATIVE SWEETENERS

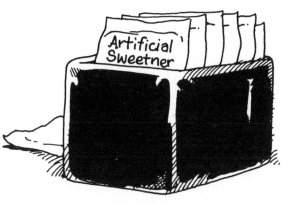

Alternative sweeteners may be classified as "non-nutritive sweeteners" or "nutritive sweeteners." A non-nutritive sweetener is a product that does not contain calories. The term "nutritive sweetener" on a label refers to a product that contains calories.

Non-nutritive Sweeteners

Non-nutritive sweeteners are usually intensely sweet. Although some of these products contain calories, they are usually used in such small quantities that they do not make a significant contribution to caloric intake. Two examples are saccharin and aspartame.

Saccharin: Although saccharin has been used for about 80 years in the United States, in 1977 it was designated by the FDA as a potential carcinogen or co-carcinogen. A two-generation male rat study showed a probability of inducing cancer with increased use of very large doses of saccharin. However, there is no substantial evidence to suggest it causes cancers in humans when used in expected and reasonable amounts. The policy of the American Diabetes Association is that, in light of current evidence, there are no indications for individuals with diabetes to avoid using saccharin.

Aspartame: Aspartame is a combination of two amino acids (aspartic acid and phenylalanine) that is about 200 times sweeter than sucrose. Although technically it is a nutritive sweetener because it provides four calories per gram, there is only .1 calorie in the amount of aspartame necessary to produce the same sweetness as one teaspoon of sugar, and so it is usually classed with the non-nutritive sweeteners.

Aspartame is marketed as a tabletop sweetener called Equal®. It is found in food products under the brand name NutraSweet®. Aspartame is broken down in the body in a manner similar to protein, but it can be harmful to people with a rare inherited metabolic abnormality called phenylketonuria or PKU. A warning to people with PKU appears on packages of Equal and products sweetened with NutraSweet. Equal is available in single serving packets and tablets. One packet is as sweet as 2 teaspoons of sugar (32 calories) but supplies only 4 calories. Each tablet is as sweet as one teaspoon of sugar but contributes only 1/4 the calories.

Equal can be used to sweeten foods and beverages in which you would normally use table sugar. Use it in simple recipes that do not require heating, because Equal loses sweetness when exposed to heat. In addition, Equal does not provide the necessary bulk and structure required in home-baked foods such as cakes, breads, and cookies.

The high heat needed for home canning will cause Equal to lose its sweetness, but jams, jellies, fruit butters and other preserves can be made with it for freezer storage.

Questions concerning the safety of aspartame have been raised. Aspartame underwent more than 100 scientific studies to establish its safety. Various safety concerns raised during the 16 years of aspartame's development and approval were addressed by the FDA. In each case, the FDA concluded that the various safety concerns raised were not supported by scientific evidence.

One of the issues raised is that in the body, aspartame breaks down rapidly into methanol, which the critics say is harmful to the person consuming it. To understand why this is not so, consider this: If the average daily amount of sugar consumed by a person in the United States were replaced by aspartame, which would be virtually impossible to do because sugar is our leading food additive, it would produce 280 milligrams of phenylalanine, 226 milligrams of aspartic acid, and 54 milligrams of methanol. These amounts of phenylalanine and aspartic acid are less than the quantities provided by 6 ounces of milk or 3 ounces of beef. The same amount of methanol is provided by 8 ounces of fruit or vegetable juice or 2 ounces of gin. As you can see, many foods such as fruit, fruit juices, tomato juice, vegetable soup, and alcohol all break down into methanol. The methanol from the breakdown of aspartame is the same as the methanol produced in the human body from food.

Another issue raised is that phenylalanine, one of the two primary components of aspartame, can cause changes in the brain's chemistry and result in behavioral changes, particularly in children. At expected levels of intake, phenylalanine levels do not exceed those observed after normal meals. Even at abusive intake levels, the amount of phenylalanine in the blood is below amounts expected to show toxic effects. A panel convened by the FDA concluded that the evidence did not support the charge that aspartame might harm the brain, but they did recommend that long-term animal studies be conducted.

The FDA has concluded that an acceptable daily intake of aspartame is up to 50 milligrams per kilogram (2.2 pounds) of body weight. If all sugar in the average person's diet were replaced with aspartame, the resulting intake would be 34 milligrams per kilogram. A 12-ounce can of diet soda contains approximately 150 to 200 milligrams of aspartame, which is less than 3 milligrams per kilogram for a 150-pound person.

Studies have found no evidence of adverse effects even at levels of aspartame consumption six times greater than what 99 percent of the general public could be expected to consume. All of this has led various health groups and agencies to conclude that aspartame appears to meet our expectations for a safe, low-calorie sweetener with no undesirable aftertaste.

Nutritive Sweeteners

Nutritive sweeteners are caloric sweeteners identical in caloric values on a weight basis to sucrose. Therefore, they do not serve as an alternative to sucrose in terms of calories. Various nutritive sweeteners are defined in Chapter 32.

Fructose, sorbitol and other sugar alcohols fall in this category. Sugar alcohols are synthetic products made from "ose" sugars. Fructose and sorbitol have been used in Western Europe as alternatives to glucose-containing sweeteners such as sucrose. Although they may be more slowly digested and absorbed, they still contribute calories, and therefore must be counted in the diabetic meal plan.

Fructose: Fructose is a commercial sugar considerably sweeter than sucrose, although its sweetness actually depends on how it is used in cooking. If used in products that are cold and acidic in nature, it is sweeter. If used in products that require heat, such as baking, it is usually not sweeter than sucrose. Fructose is suitable for baking, canning and freezing.

In persons with diabetes who have adequate insulin available, fructose causes a more modest increase in blood glucose levels than other simple sugars. However, use of fructose is not recommended in persons with poorly-controlled diabetes with an insulin deficiency, because fructose is readily converted to glucose. It is also equal to sucrose in caloric value and so must be restricted in obese individuals and used as part of total caloric restrictions.

Sorbitol: Sorbitol is the most commonly used sugar alcohol. It is readily converted to fructose and metabolized through the same pathway. One of the major problems with sorbitol is the laxative effect it has on the gastrointestinal tract. Many food products sweetened with sorbitol end up with more calories than the product they are replacing because of added fat used to make the sorbitol soluble.

The following table can help you use alternative sweeteners successfully!

A Handy Guide to *Sweetening Without Sugar*

Type of Sweetener and Brand Name	Major Sweetening Ingredient	Sweetness Compared to Sugar Amt. Sweetener = Amt. Sugar	Manufacturer's Suggested Uses
Non-Nutritive (few or no calories)			
• EQUAL® packets and EQUAL SWEET TABS®	Aspartame	1 packet = 2 tsp. 1 tablet = 1 tsp.	Table use and added to cold or hot foods.
• SUCARYL® liquid • SWEET 10® liquid • NUTRADIET® liquid	Saccharin	1/8 tsp. (10 drops) = 1 tsp. 3/8 tsp. = 1 Tbsp. 2 Tbsp. = 1 cup	Table use and in cooking.
• SUGAR TWIN,® regular and brown sugar replacement, powder and packet • SPRINKLE SWEET® packet	Saccharin	1 tsp. = 1 tsp. 1 Tbsp. = 1 Tbsp. 1 cup = 1 cup 1 packet = 2 tsp.	Baking, cooking, and table use.
• SWEET 'N LOW,® regular and brown sugar replacement, powder and packet	Saccharin	1 tsp. = 1/4 cup 1-1/3 tsp. = 1/3 cup 2 tsp. = 1/2 cup 4 tsp. = 1 cup 1 packet = 2 tsp.	Baking, cooking, canning, and table use.
• FEATHERWEIGHT® tablets (1/4 grain)	Saccharin	1 tablet = 1 tsp.	Table use.
Nutritive (contains calories)			
• Fructose, powder and packet	Fructose	1 tsp. = 12 calories and 3 grams carbohydrate 1 packet = 1 tsp. fructose powder	Table use and in cooking, tastes sweeter in cold foods.

Chapter Thirty-Four
CANNING AND FREEZING

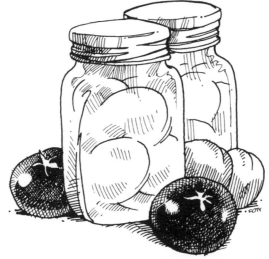

Pride and pleasure can be yours when home-grown produce or in-season fruit market specials are preserved. Canning and freezing are easy and safe if you follow instructions carefully. Use these hints to adapt your favorite recipes for your meal plan.

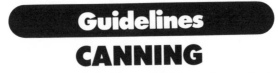

Guidelines

CANNING

In canning, heat is applied to a food in order to destroy microorganisms (yeasts, molds, bacteria) and to halt enzyme activity which causes food to spoil.

The acidity of a food is one factor to consider when deciding on a method of canning. Acid occurring naturally in foods has the ability to destroy most bacteria. Therefore, a high acid food can be preserved using a lower heat treatment, such as a boiling water bath. Low acid foods need the pressure canning process. High acid fruits and vegetables include apples, berries, cherries, peaches, rhubarb and tomatoes. Low acid vegetables include asparagus, beans, beets, carrots, corn, potatoes and squash.

In the water bath method for high acid fruits and vegetables, food is packed into jars and covered with a hot cooking solution. Jars are placed on a rack and quickly lowered into water. There should be two inches of water above the jars. Begin counting process time as soon as water in the canner reaches a rolling boil. Cover the canner and process with the water boiling for the recommended length of time.

Pressure canning methods should be used for low acid foods. Follow the manufacturer's directions for using pressure canners.

Packing methods include hot pack, raw or cold pack. Hot-packed food is heated thoroughly before packing. In hot packing, place fruit in a large kettle and cook until tender. Taste the cooked product and add sweetening, lemon juice or spices as needed. The hot fruit is then packed into hot, clean jars, liquid is added to within one-half inch of jar rim, lids are added, and the jar is boiled in the water bath. Hot-packing is good for fruits that tend to discolor and is also used for many vegetables. Raw-packing food saves time in the canning process and in some cases helps retain flavor and food value. In the raw or cold pack method fruit is placed directly into hot, clean jars, liquid is added to within one-half inch from top of jar, jar lids are screwed on, and the jar is placed into a boiling water bath or pressure cooker to process. Liquid must be added to the fruit to help the cooking process.

When cooling the jars, place them upright on dry surfaces. Let jars cool for 12 hours, then check seals. If the center of the lid holds down when pressed and the lid does not move, the jar is sealed.

Use your canned foods within one year. When opening canned food, carefully inspect the contents for signs of spoilage. Look for cloudy liquid, an "off" odor, bulging lids, deterioration or patches of mold. Never taste doubtful food! Home canned low acid foods should be boiled for 10 to 15 minutes before serving.

Sugar is not needed in the canning process to prevent spoilage. It is often added to fruits to help hold shape, color and flavor. Fruits may be easily canned without added sugar if they are canned in their own juice or water. Processing time is the same for unsweetened fruit as for sweetened. Some of the manufacturers of artificial sweeteners have guidelines for using their products in canning. Artificial sweeteners added to the canning process may produce a bitter taste. You can add an artificial sweetener at serving time if you like.

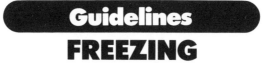

Guidelines

FREEZING

Fresh fruits no longer know a season. With proper freezing procedures, you can capture the beauty, texture and taste of products from gardens and orchards.

Choose fruits that are in their prime, ripe and firm. Prepare fruits for the way you plan to use them by peeling or slicing them.

For fruits that tend to discolor, you can add lemon juice, ascorbic acid or a compound containing ascorbic acid, such as Fruit Fresh.

Fruits are sometimes packed with sugar or syrups when frozen to add texture and flavor. This is not necessary to prevent spoilage; fruits can be packed unsweetened. (Some fruits can also be packed dry without adding liquid.) A syrup for freezing may be made from an artificial sweetener and water. The syrup should completely cover the fruit when it is used. Follow the manufacturer's directions for the amount of artificial sweetener to add to avoid a bitter taste. In addition, fruit can be artificially sweetened before serving.

Fruits and vegetables stored at 0° F or below will maintain high quality for 8 to 12 months. However, unsweetened fruit tends to lose quality more rapidly, so include these foods in your menus as soon as feasible.

Tips On Preserving Without Sugar

Barbara Larson of Montevideo, Minnesota, has shared her experience with freezing and canning fruits, jams and jellies without sugar. She exhibits her canned products at fairs and consistently wins ribbons for excellence! The following suggestions are hers.

For canning fruits, use the water bath method and artificially sweetened syrup. Then process the fruit the same as fruit canned in sugar syrup. Pack peaches, pears and apricots raw in pint jars; add boiling water or syrup to cover the fruit; wipe off the jar rim; place a lid and ring on firmly; and process the jar for 25 minutes in a boiling water bath. For pears and peaches, add one teaspoon of an ascorbic acid type fruit freshener (such as Fruit Fresh) per pint of syrup to keep the fruit from darkening.

Prepare plums and cherries the same way. Prick them instead of removing the pits. The process time is 20 minutes for pint jars. Plums, if fully ripe when canned, are fine in a water pack. The other fruits seem more flavorful when canned in an artificially sweetened syrup. Make the syrup with one tablespoon liquid sweetener for each pint of boiling water. Pour the syrup into the jars while it is boiling hot.

Put hot unsweetened applesauce into pint jars and process for 25 minutes in a boiling water bath. The sweetness of applesauce depends on the variety and ripeness of the apple. Ripe Beacon and Cortland apples need no sweetening. Sweetener can be added to applesauce just before serving. Check the jars when they are cool to make sure the lids are sealed. Store them in a cool place.

Fruits can also be canned without sugar using a syrup made from fruit juice. When using the canned fruit with the juice, be aware there is carbohydrate in the juice as well as the fruit. One-half cup fruit and juice equals one fruit exchange; one-half cup fruit with one third cup of juice equals two fruit exchanges.

To make the syrup use:

> 1/3 cup orange juice
> 4 cups liquified fruit
> (peach, pear, etc., pureed in blender)
> 1½ cups white grape juice (Catawba)
> 7¾ cups water

Cook for five minutes at boiling and then reduce heat. Pour it over fruit and process canned fruit in a boiling water bath for 30 minutes.

Or make the following syrup and follow the same procedure.

> 10 cups water
> 1/3 cup orange juice
> 1½ cups white grape juice (Catawba)

Raspberries, strawberries and cantaloupe balls or chunks can be frozen without sugar or syrup. Use small containers that hold no more than a cup. There is some vitamin loss in freezing them "dry," but it is well worth the loss to have the color and flavor of these fruits available during the winter months.

Tasty sugarless jams and jellies can also be made from fruit. Use Slim Set, which is a pectin that requires no sugar, to help the fruit or juice to gel. Simple directions are enclosed in the Slim Set package. Slim Set Jelling Mix contributes 3.2 calories and 0.7 grams of carbohydrate to one serving (one tablespoon) of jam or jelly, prepared as directed in the instructions. The total amount of calories and carbohydrate in a Slim Set jam or jelly depends on the type of fruit and sweetener used in making the batch. Jellies are made from four cups of juice. Jams are made with three cups of crushed fruit and one cup of water. Use the amount of artificial sweetener equivalent to 1/2 or 3/4 cup sugar per batch. DO NOT substitute artificial sweetener for sugar in a regular jam or jelly recipe, it will be oversweet and taste very bitter.

Grape, apple, pineapple, cranberry and orange jellies can be made using the purchased unsweetened juices, either canned or frozen. You can also make your own apple, crabapple, cherry and grape juice for jelly. Delicious jams can be made in these flavors: peach, pear, apricot, apricot-pineapple, peach-plum, sour pie cherry, raspberry and strawberry. When making jam with light colored fruits, add two teaspoons of Fruit Fresh to retain the bright color.

Pour hot jam or jelly into half-pint jars up to 1/8″ from the top; wipe off the jar rim; put the lid and ring on securely; and tip the jar upside down for about 10 minutes. Then turn the jars right-side-up and let them cool. In almost all cases they seal this way. If one does not happen to seal, refrigerate it and use it in season. Store the sealed jars in a cool dark place. Enjoy!

Chapter Thirty-Five
ADDING FIBER
TO YOUR MEAL PLAN

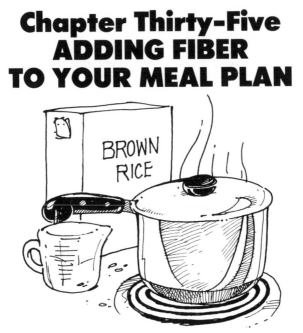

Foods from grains are often referred to as fattening, but this description is not really warranted. Remember, ounce for ounce, fat has more than twice as many calories as protein or carbohydrate. These are not "fattening" foods unless they are consumed in excess, since they are low in fat, moderate in protein, and high in carbohydrates.

What makes these foods fattening are the high-calorie sauces, cream, dressings, and spreads added to foods containing fiber. Examples are sour cream on baked potatoes, gravy on brown rice, butter or margarine on whole wheat breads. An average slice of bread contains only about 80 calories. Adding a tablespoon of honey, preserves, or butter doubles the calories!

Whole grains such as barley, bran, brown rice, buckwheat grouts (kasha), bulgur (cracked wheat), cornmeal, popcorn, whole wheat, and wheat germ supply protein, B vitamins, and iron along with being excellent sources of fiber in the diet. Try experimenting with a variety of fibers:

Barley.—Although the outer hull has been removed from barley, the kernel still contains the endosperm which is mostly protein, the bean, which contains B vitamins, and the germ or sprouting section which contains fiber, making barley a nutritious food.

Bran flakes or unprocessed bran.—Bran by itself resembles fine sawdust in taste and texture and so is not consumed right from the box. Instead it is added to other food products or used in baking or cooking.

Brown rice.—The whole unpolished rice grain with only the outer hull (or husk) and a small portion of the bran removed. Its color comes from the outer layer of nutritious, fiber-rich bran. it has a slightly nutty flavor and a chewier texture than white rice.

Buckwheat Groats.—Buckwheat seeds are called groats, and cooked or roasted groats are called kasha.

Bulgur.—Whole wheat berry that is parboiled, dried, and broken up. It cooks quickly in only 5 to 10 minutes.

Cornmeal.—Ground corn, also call polenta.

Couscous.—Precooked hard-cracked granules of semolina wheat. They can be cooked quickly by a soak-and-steam method, or with a couscousiere, a steamer made specifically for couscous.

Whole grain flours.—Whole wheat, rye, cracked wheat, buckwheat, and stone ground.

Legume.—"Legume" is a general term referring to dried beans, peas, and lentils. Start with lentils, split peas, and lima beans—these are the most easily digested legumes. Begin with small servings to give your body a chance to adjust.

Oats.—Oat grain closely resembles a kernel of wheat in structure. Unlike wheat, the nutritious bran and germ are not removed in processing because oats are not refined. They are an excellent source of soluble fibers, which give oatmeal a gummy texture. Oats contain a natural preservative that gives them and products made from them a longer shelf life.

Popcorn.—Popcorn kernels have more hard starch then other types of corn, which helps them to "explode" when heated. Popcorn is an excellent snack food.

Rye.—Usually used as a flour. Color is the clue to nutritional value. Light and medium rye flours have been sifted (bolted), which removes much of the nutritious bran; dark rye flour is unbolted and far more nourishing. Most of the bread called "rye bread" in the United States is made with flour that is less than one-third rye flour.

Wheat germ.—The vitamin-and-mineral rich wheat embryo that is separated out when flour is refined. It is a tasty, nourishing supplement that can be added to all kinds of recipes—breads, casseroles, breadings, etc. Because it contains wheat-germ oil, it should be stored in the refrigerator after the jar is opened.

Wild rice.—Not really rice but the seed of an aquatic grass that is native to America. The whole grain is cooked and it is never refined.

Cooking Methods

Whole wheat or whole grain flour.—Whole wheat flour spoils rapidly and should be stored in a cool, dry place to prevent spoilage; store it in a freezer or refrigerator. Because whole-wheat flour is bulkier than white flour, you'll need to make adjustments when baking with it. For each cup of white flour called for in a recipe, you can substitute:

- One cup whole-wheat flour minus 2 tablespoons. Decrease the amount of oil called for in the recipe by 1 tablespoon and increase the liquid by 1 or 2 tablespoons. (This is not necessary if a finely ground whole wheat flour is used.)
- Or use 3/4 cup white flour plus either 1/4 cup wheat germ or 1/4 cup bran.
- Or use 1/2 cup white flour and 1/2 cup whole wheat flour.

Whole grains.—Most whole grains require more cooking time than the refined grains. When cooking grain, follow these steps: Rinse the grain in cold water and drain well. Bring water to a boil (stock or milk may be used instead). Slowly pour grain into water, stirring constantly. Let the water come to a boil again and turn the heat down to the lowest possible temperature. Cook slowly until all the water is absorbed.

If you have cooked the grain the full time and it still seems hard or tough, add a little boiling water, cover and continue cooking. Do not stir it any more than absolutely necessary or it will be gummy. Be sure not to lift the cover while the grain is cooking—steam will escape and the grain might stick.

Brown rice.—When cooking brown rice, remember to first wash the raw rice well and drain. Place it in a saucepan with enough room for the rice to triple in volume. Add twice the amount of boiling water as rice and return to boil. Cover and reduce heat to the lowest possible setting. Let rice cook very slowly for 45 minutes. Do not stir; stirring makes rice pasty. Remove the rice from heat and let it stand several minutes. This will steam the rice and dry it even more. Don't add salt until after the rice is cooked; salt tends to harden the kernels.

For a slightly different taste, before cooking, stir the washed rice in a dry saucepan over medium heat until the grain is dry and lightly toasted. This will enhance the nutty flavor.

Bulgur.—Bulgur can be eaten uncooked by soaking it in water for several hours. It doubles its dry volume upon cooking or soaking. Do not wash bulgur before, nor rise after cooking. Do not lift the lid while bulgur is cooking. It does not need to be stirred. Bulgur continues to expand (swell) even after cooking time as long as moisture is available. It may be cooked and stored in the refrigerator for future use.

Couscous.—To cook couscous, place it in a bowl and pour water over it (1½ cups couscous to 3 cups water). Let sit for 10 to 15 minutes until the water is absorbed. The couscous will now be soft; fluff it with a fork or with your hands. Place the couscous in a colander, sieve, or the top part of a couscousiere, above the cooking liquid, making sure the bottom of the colander does not touch the liquid. Seal off the space between the colander and the pot with a towel or cheesecloth. Cover and bring the liquid to a boil. Let steam for 10 minutes, then remove the couscous from the pot and place in a large bowl. Adjust the seasonings and serve at once.

Kasha.—Uncooked groats are commonly mixed with a beaten egg or egg white and then cooked briefly over high heat for 2 minutes in a skillet. This keeps the groats from sticking together when cooked further in liquid. When dry-roasting stir constantly to separate the kernels and keep them from burning. Then add 2 cups of boiling liquid (water or broth) for each cup of groats, cover the pot, and cook the kasha over a low heat for about 10 to 15 minutes until the liquid is absorbed.

Wild rice.—The darker the rice the longer it will take to cook. Cook until most of the grains curl and pop, approximately 45 minutes to 1 hour. Do not overcook wild rice or it will be soft and lose its texture.

Cooking Times and Proportions for Dinner Grains

Grain (1 cup dry measure)	Water	Cooking Time	Yield
Barley	3 cups	1 hr.	3½ cups
Brown Rice	2 cups	45-50 min.	3 cups
Bulgur*	2 cups	15 min.	2½ cups
Cracked Wheat	2 cups	25 min.	2⅓ cups
Kasha	2 cups	15 min.	2½ cups
Millet	3 cups	30-40 min.	3½ cups
Coarse Corn Meal (Polenta)	4 cups	25 min.	3 cups
Wild Rice	3 cups	1 hr. or more	4 cups

*Bulgur can also be prepared by soaking in warm water for about 1 hour, eliminating the need for cooking.

Legumes (Dried Beans, Peans, Lentils)

Beans, peas, and lentils are some of the best sources of fiber and are full of protein. However, when eaten by themselves, they are "incomplete proteins." That is, they lack or are low in certain amino acids needed by the body. There are nine amino acids that cannot be made by the body and must come from food. Most beans (except soybeans) are deficient in two of these amino acids. Whole wheat, whole grains, nuts, seeds, and dairy products, which are rich in these two amino acids, should be combined with legumes in order to receive complete protein in your diet if you substitute legumes for meat. See Chapter Nine for more information on vegetarian diets.

Legumes may be hard for the body to digest and can cause flatulence (intestinal gas) if you are not used to eating them. It is best to start with lentils, split peas, or lima beans because they are more easily digested. Begin with small servings to give your body a chance to adjust and to allow a gradual change in the intestinal flora.

Beans

Before cooking beans, make sure you rinse and sort them thoroughly, as they come directly from the fields. To cut cooking time, soak all beans overnight. (Soybeans should be refrigerated during soaking to prevent fermentation.) Another method is to put beans and water in a pot, bring the water to a boil, simmer for two minutes, then remove from heat and allow to stand covered for one hour. Also, don't mix different kinds of beans when cooking unless you are using a crockpot. Cover beans with water, bring them to a boil and let them simmer until tender. Keep beans covered with liquid at all times during cooking. Check occasionally and add more water if needed. Don't add salt, oil, or spices until beans are tender, or they won't cook. Keep the pot partially covered at all times; beans usually boil over if covered tightly. If you're cooking beans for a salad or any dish where they should be firm, cook just until tender. For soups, beans may be cooked much longer.

Time Savers

- Cook large batches and freeze in serving size portions.
- Use a crockpot for cooking beans. A mixture of beans may be cooked in the same pot.
- Use canned beans. Check labels and try to avoid those canned with sugar or rinse off the beans before use to remove added salt and sugar.
- Instead of overnight soaking, bring the legumes and water to a boil, simmer for 2 minutes, remove from heat and allow to stand for 1 hour.

- Pressure cooking can be an advantage with legumes because of shortness in cooking times. It also yields a more tender bean. Place the beans in water equal to three or four times their volume and bring to a boil in the pressure cooker. Cover and bring them to 15 pounds pressure, cook most beans 20 to 25 minutes and lentils and split peas 10 to 15 minutes. Cool the pressure cooker immediately under cold running water. Open the cooker and drain the stock from the beans.

Cooking Times and Proportions for Beans

Beans (1 cup dry measure)	Water	Cooking Time	Yield
Black beans	4 cups	1½-2 hrs.	2 cups
Black-eyed peas	3 cups	1-2 hrs.	2 cups
Garbanzos	4 cups	3-4 hrs.	2 cups
Great Northern beans	3½ cups	2 hrs.	2 cups
Kidney beans	3 cups	1½ hrs.	2 cups
Lentils and split peas	3 cups	1 hrs.	2¼ cups
Lima	2 cups	1½ hrs.	1¼ cups
Baby lima	2 cups	1½ hrs.	1¾ cups
Pinto beans	3 cups	2-2½ hrs.	2 cups
Small red beans	3 cups	3 hrs.	2 cups
Small white beans (navy, etc.)	3 cups	1½ hrs.	2 cups
Soybeans	4 cups	2-3 or more hrs.	2 cups
Soy grits	2 cups	15-20 minutes	2 cups

Foods containing fiber contribute valuable nutrients along with the every-increasing discoveries of their health benefits, making this food of yesterday an exciting and essential part of eating today.

Chapter Thirty-Six
CALCULATING EXCHANGES
FROM YOUR FAVORITE RECIPES

If you have recipes that you enjoy and use often, you may wish to convert them to exchanges. The following steps will help:

1. List all the ingredients in the recipe and their amounts.

2. Identify the exchange group and record the number of exchanges in each ingredient. Refer to the table below — Commonly Used Ingredients — Approximate Exchanges.

3. Total each exchange group.

4. Divide the total number of exchanges for each group by the number of servings in the recipe and round off to the nearest 1/2 exchange. Anything less than 1/2 need not be counted.

The following table gives the approximate exchange values of ingredients commonly used for baking and cooking.

Commonly Used Ingredients — Approximate Exchanges

Food Item	Amount	Carbo-hydrate (Gms)	Protein (Gms)	Fat (Gms)	Exchanges
Biscuit mix	1/2 cup	37	4	8	2½ starch/bread 1 fat
Bread crumbs	1 cup	65	11	4	4 starch/bread
Cake flour, sifted	1 cup	79	8	1	5 starch/bread
Graham cracker crumbs	1 cup	90	8	14	6 starch/bread 2 fat

Food Item	Amount	Carbo-hydrate (Gms)	Protein (Gms)	Fat (Gms)	Exchanges
Chow Mein noodles	1/2 cup	17	3	8	1 starch/bread 1½ fat
Cornmeal (uncooked)	1 cup	117	11	5	7½ starch/bread
Cornstarch	2 Tbsp.	14	—	—	1 starch/bread
Cream soups, undiluted	1 can	20	3	18	1 starch/bread 3½ fat
Flour					
all purpose, unsifted	1 cup	87	11	1	6 starch/bread
whole wheat, unsifted	1 cup	80	16	2	5 starch/bread
rye, medium	1 cup	66	10	2	4½ starch/bread
Macaroni					
uncooked (3½ oz.)	1 cup	79	7	Trace	5 starch/bread
cooked	1 cup	41	7	1	3 starch/bread
Noodles					
egg, uncooked (2½ oz.)	1 cup	59	7	1	4 starch/bread
cooked	1 cup	40	8	3	2½ starch/bread
Oatmeal, uncooked	1 cup	54	15	6	3½ starch/bread 1 fat
Rice, white & brown					
uncooked	1/4 cup	39	3	—	2½ starch/bread
cooked	1 cup	36	3	1	2½ starch/bread
Wild, uncooked	1/4 cup	21	4	—	1½ starch/bread
Long grain, instant, dry	1/4 cup	26	2	—	2 starch/bread
Long grain, instant, cooked	1 cup	40	4	—	2½ starch/bread
Spaghetti					
uncooked (3½ oz.)	1 cup	79	7	Trace	5 starch/bread
cooked	1 cup	41	'7	1	2½ starch/bread
Wheat germ	1/4 cup (1 oz.)	13	9	3	1 starch/bread 1 lean meat

Food Item	Amount	Carbo-hydrate (Gms)	Protein (Gms)	Fat (Gms)	Exchanges
Dairy Products					
Butter or margarine	1/4 cup or 1/2 stick	—	—	49	10 fat
	1/2 cup or 1 stick	—	—	98	20 fat
Cheese, cheddar, grated	1 cup	2	29	37	4 med. fat meat 3 fat
cream	4 oz.	3	8	40	1 med. fat meat 7 fat
mozzarella, grated	1 cup	3	28	18	4 med. fat meat
Parmesan, grated	1/4 cup	1	8	6	1 med. fat meat
Cream					
half & half	1/2 cup	5	3	14	3 fat
sour half & half	1/2 cup	5	3	14	3 fat
sour	1/2 cup	4	3	20	5 fat
sour, imitation	1/2 cup	8	3	23	1/2 starch/bread 4½ fat
heavy, unwhipped	1/4 cup	2	1	22	4 fat
heavy, whipped	1/2 cup	2	1	22	4 fat
Egg yolk	1 medium	—	3	5	1 fat
Egg, whole	1 medium	—	6	6	1 med. fat meat
Milk					
condensed, sweetened	1/3 cup	54	8	9	1 skim milk 3 fruit 2 fat
evaporated, whole	1/2 cup	12	8	10	1 skim milk 2 fat
evaporated, skim	1/2 cup	14	9	—	1 skim milk
nonfat dry solids, instant	1 cup	31	21	—	2½ skim milk
Yogurt, plain low fat	1 cup	13	9	1	1 skim milk

Food Item	Amount	Carbo-hydrate (Gms)	Protein (Gms)	Fat (Gms)	Exchanges
Fats, Oils, Chocolate and Cocoa					
Chocolate, bitter	1 oz.	7	4	16	1/2 starch/bread 3 fat
Chocolate flavored syrup	2 Tbsp.	17	1	1	1 fruit
Chocolate chips					
Real chocolate	1 cup (6 oz.)	105	8	48	7 fruit 10 fat
Chocolate flavored	1 cup (6 oz.)	106	10	48	7 fruit 10 fat
Carob powder or carob flour	1 cup	113	6	2	7½ starch/bread
Cocoa powder	4 Tbsp.	16	6	2	1 starch/bread
Mayonnaise	1/2 cup	1	1	88	17½ fat
Mayonnaise type salad dressing	1/2 cup	14	1	55	1 starch/bread 11 fat
Olives, sliced	1/2 cup	2	1	9	2 fat
Shortening	1/2 cup	—	—	111	22 fat
	1 cup	—	—	221	44 fat
Vegetable oils	1/2 cup	—	—	111	22 fat
	1 cup	—	—	221	44 fat
Fruits and Vegetables					
Barbecue sauce (average)	3 Tbsp.	15	0	1	1 fruit
Catsup or chili sauce	1/2 cup	30	2	1	2 starch/bread **or** 3 fruit
Dates	1 cup	130	4	1	8½ fruit
Raisins	1/2 cup	55	2	—	3½ fruit
Tomatoes **or** tomato juice	1 cup	9	2	—	1/2 starch/bread **or** 2 vegetable
Tomato sauce or puree	1 cup	20	4	1	1 starch/bread **or** 4 vegetable

Food Item	Amount	Carbo-hydrate (Gms)	Protein (Gms)	Fat (Gms)	Exchanges
Sugars and Syrups					
Corn syrup	1 cup	242	—	—	16 fruit
Gelatin dessert (Jell-O)	3 oz. box	74	6	—	2 starch/bread 3 fruit
Honey	1 cup	264	1	—	17½ fruit
Molasses					
light	1 cup	213	—	—	14 fruit
dark	1 cup	180	—	—	12 fruit
Sugar					
brown, packed	1 cup	212	—	—	14 fruit
powdered, sifted	1 cup	100	—	—	6½ fruit
powdered, unsifted	1 cup	119	—	—	8 fruit
white	1 cup	199	—	—	13 fruit
Nuts and Miscellaneous					
Almonds	1/2 cup	15	14	41	1 starch/bread 1½ med. fat meat 6½ fat
Cashew nuts	1 cup	29	17	46	2 starch/bread 1½ med. fat meat 7½ fat
Coconut, dried, shredded	1 cup	33	2	24	2 fruit 5 fat
Peanut butter	1 cup	34	76	137	10 med. fat meat 17 fat
Peanuts	1 oz.	5	7	14	1 med. fat meat 2 fat
Pecans	1 cup	13	9	73	1 starch/bread 1 med. fat meat 13½ fat
Sunflower seeds, shelled	3½ oz.	21	25	56	1½ starch/bread 3 med. fat meat 8 fat
Walnuts	1 cup	16	15	64	1 starch/bread 2 med. fat meat 10½ fat

Food Item	Amount	Carbo-hydrate (Gms)	Protein (Gms)	Fat (Gms)	Exchanges
Meats					
Chicken, canned, boned	5½ oz.	—	34	18	5 lean meat
Ground beef, lean	1 lb. raw **or** 11 oz. cooked	—	79	66	11 med. fat meat 2 fat
Salmon, pink	16 oz. can, 13 oz. drained		93	27	13 lean meat
Tuna, water packed	6½ oz.		53	3	7½ lean meat (subtract 4 fat)
Tuna, packed in oil	6½ oz.		45	30	6 med. fat meat

Here are two examples of recipes that have been converted into exchanges. Also given is a sample form for you to use with your favorite recipe.

Sesame Cookie — Yield: 24 cookies

Ingredients	Starch/ Bread	Meat	Veg.	Fruit	Milk	Fat	Free
2 Tbsp. sesame seed							FREE
2 cups sifted flour	12						
1/4 teaspoon salt							FREE
1/2 cup butter or margarine						20	
1/4 cup shortening						11	
1 cup sugar				13			
1 egg		1					
1 teaspoon vanilla extract							FREE
Total Exchanges	12	1	0	13	0	31	
Total Exchanges / Total Servings = Exchanges per serving	1/2	1/24	0	1/2	0	1	

1 Sesame Cookie (1 serving) = 1/2 starch/bread, 1/2 fruit, 1 fat exchange.

Tuna Party Casserole — Yield: 4 Servings (1 cup each)

Ingredients	Starch/ Bread	Meat	Veg.	Fruit	Milk	Fat	Free
4 Tbsp. margarine						10	
1/2 cup onions			1				
1/4 cup chopped green peppers							FREE
4 cups cooked noodles	10						
1½ teaspoons salt							FREE
1/2 teaspoon pepper							FREE
1 can cream of mushroom soup	1					3½	
1 No. 2 can tomatoes, drained			4				
6½ oz. water packed tuna		7½				-4	
1/4 teaspoon thyme							FREE
1 cup (1 oz.) crushed potato chips	1					2	
Total Exchanges	12	7½	5	0	0	12	
Total Exchanges / Total Servings = Exchanges per serving	3	2	1	0	0	3	

1 cup Tuna Party Casserole = 3 starch/bread, 2 lean meat, 1 vegetable, 3 fat exchanges.

Your Recipe: _____

Ingredients	Exchanges						
	Starch/ Bread	Meat	Veg.	Fruit	Milk	Fat	Free
Total Exchanges							

$$\frac{\text{Total Exchanges}}{\text{Total Servings}} = \text{Exchanges per serving}$$

Chapter Thirty-Seven
RECIPE MODIFICATIONS FOR LOWERING FAT AND INCREASING FIBER

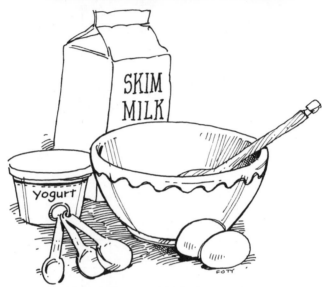

You can modify recipes to reduce calories, total fat, saturated fat, cholesterol, sodium and/or concentrated sweets. The two basic ways to modify a recipe are to change a cooking technique or to change an ingredient. An example of changing a cooking technique would be to saute vegetables in broth instead of oil or butter, thus reducing total fat as well as possibly the type of fat. You can modify ingredients by reducing them, eliminating them completely, or by substituting a more acceptable ingredient.

To reduce an ingredient, analyze the function of the ingredient in a recipe. Is it a necessary part of the final product, such as sugar in a cake? If so, you may not be able to eliminate the ingredient completely. But you may be able to reduce the amount used. Products that can be eliminated are those added for appearance or because of habit and tradition. These products may be high in sodium or sugar.

Many substitutions can be made in recipes to lower the fat and cholesterol content. While taste and texture may change, the results are often just as pleasing. Remember—"The proof of the pudding is in the eating."

Possible substitutions to consider are:

- **Evaporated skim milk for cream.** However, in order to whip evaporated skim milk it must be partially frozen.

- **Skim milk for whole milk.**

- **Egg substitutes for whole eggs.** However, some egg substitutes may have objectionable flavors. Flavor extracts may help disguise them. Using two egg whites in place of one egg is another possibility.

- **Margarine for butter.** However, soft or tub margarines will not cream. Diet margarines contain more water and less fat and cannot be substituted ounce-per-ounce for butter.

- **Oils for hydrogenated fats (shortening).** However, crusts may not have the same flakiness, and dough may stick to rolling pins. Oils will not cream. One cup of shortening can be replaced by 3/4 cup of oil; 1/2 cup shortening by 1/3 cup of oil.

- **Cocoa plus oil for chocolate.** However, cocoa will not solidify to form a coating.

- **Whole grains for refined ones.**

- **Reduce amount of sugar in recipes.** Sugar and other sweeteners add flavor, color, tenderness and crispness in baked products. In many recipes you can reduce the amount of sugar called for by at least 1/3 to 1/2 without affecting the quality of product. A helpful guideline: use no more than 1/4 cup of added sweetener (sugar, honey, molasses, etc.) per one cup of flour. Adding extra vanilla will enhance the sweetness of a recipe. Vanilla, cinnamon and nutmeg all give the illusion of sweetness without adding calories.

Persons with diabetes will generally enjoy their food products the most when they use regular foods and learn to substitute for them correctly in their meal plan. Sugar substitutes often do not work well, especially in baked products. Remember, just because a dessert does not contain sugar does not mean it is a "free food." The calories in the food product come from other ingredients—flour, eggs, shortening, etc.—that also produce glucose and require insulin to be metabolized as well.

Ingredient	Quantity	Substitute Recipe Modifications
Whole egg	1	1/4 cup egg substitute **or** 1 egg white + 1 tsp. vegetable oil **or** 2 egg whites
Butter	1 cup	1 cup margarine
Shortening or lard	1 cup	3/4 cup vegetable oil

Ingredient	Quantity	Substitute Recipe Modifications
Shortening	1/2 cup	1/3 cup vegetable oil
Whole milk	1 cup	1 cup skim milk
Light cream	1 cup	1 cup evaporated skim milk **or** 3 Tbsp. oil and skim milk to equal 1 cup
Heavy cream	1 cup	1 cup evaporated skim milk **or** 1 cup Poly Perx **or** 2/3 cup skim milk and 1/3 cup oil
Sour cream	1 cup	1 cup plain yogurt **or** 1 cup blended low fat cottage cheese (with lemon juice)
Regular cheese	1 oz.	1 oz. low-calorie or skim milk cheese
Flour (as thickener)	2 Tbsp.	1 Tbsp. cornstarch
Salad dressing	1 Tbsp.	1 Tbsp. low-calorie salad dressing
Baking chocolate	1 oz. (1 sq.)	3 Tbsp. powdered cocoa and 1 Tbsp. oil
Condensed soup		Homemade skim milk white sauce
Cream of celery	1 can	1 cup sauce + 1/4 cup chopped celery
Cream of chicken	1 can	1¼ cup sauce + chicken bouillon powder
Cream of mushroom	1 can	1 cup sauce + 1.4 oz. can drained mushrooms
Cream cheese		Blend 4 Tbsp. margarine with 1 cup dry low fat cottage cheese. Salt to taste. Small amount of skim milk is needed in blending.
Bacon	2 strips (1 oz.)	1 oz. lean Canadian bacon **or** 1 oz. lean ham
All-purpose white flour	1 cup	1 cup whole wheat flour minus 2 Tbsp., also decrease the amount of oil called for in the recipe by 1 Tbsp. and increase liquid by 1-2 Tbsp.; **or** 1/2 cup white + 1/2 cup whole wheat flour; **or** 3/4 cup white + 1/4 cup wheat germ and/or bran
White rice	1 cup	1 cup brown rice

Ingredient	Quantity	Substitute Recipe Modifications
Sugar		Reduce amount; reduction can be up to 1/2 to 1/3 of the original amount. Use no more than 1/4 cup of added sweetener (sugar, honey, molasses, etc.) per cup of flour.
Fat		Use no more than 1-2 Tbsp. of added oil or fat per cup of flour, compensate by increasing a low fat moist ingredient, such as buttermilk, to add moistness.
Salt		Reduce amount, try spices and herbs.

Chapter Thirty-Eight
SELECTED RECIPES

Recipes

Quick Baked Potatoe
1 large potatoe
Melted margarine, just enough to brush
   each potato half
Paprika
Parmeson Cheese   2 servings

This was not designed as a recipe book, but a few recipes especially helpful for persons with diabetes are included.

Recipe modification guidelines are included in Chapter 37 and will help you modify your favorite recipes. These guidelines help to reduce fat, sugar and calories. Chapter 36 contains guidelines to help you convert your favorite recipes into exchanges. Recipes starred (*) are from **Cooking to Stay in SHAPE.**

These first recipes can be used as delicious toppings on pancakes or French toast. Add a dab of plain low fat yogurt and you have an attractive serving.

Strawberry and Blueberry Topping*

2 cups fresh or frozen (without sugar) strawberries or blueberries

2 tsp. undiluted frozen apple juice concentrate (thawed)

Combine 1/2 cup of sliced strawberries or blueberries and 2 tsp. apple juice concentrate in a blender; process to a smooth sauce. Pour over remaining sliced strawberries or blueberries.

Yield: 4 servings   Serving size: 3/4 cup

Per serving of strawberries: Calories: 56
                              Carbohydrate: 14
                              Sodium: 1 mg.
                              Exchanges: 1 fruit

Per serving of blueberries: Calories: 64
                             Carbohydrate: 16 gms.
                             Sodium: 1 mg.
                             Exchanges: 1 fruit

Here's another topping recipe you can try. It can be used as a free food.

Maple Syrup

1¼ cups cold water   1 tsp. maple flavoring
1 Tbsp. cornstarch   1/8 tsp. salt
Artificial liquid sweetener —
   equal to 1 cup sugar

Combine ingredients in a saucepan. Bring to boil. Serve hot or cold over pancakes or waffles. Stir before using.

Yield: 1½ cups   Serving size: 1/4 cup

Per serving: Calories: 8
             Carbohydrate: 2 gms.
             Sodium: 0
             Exchanges: up to 1/2 cup free

Here is a great way to bake potatoes. The potatoes have a crispy crust and don't need any additional margarine or sour cream, thus eliminating any added fat.

Quick Baked Potato*

1 large baking potato
Melted margarine, just enough to brush each potato half
Paprika
Parmesan cheese

Cut potato in half, brush cut half with melted margarine. Sprinkle potato with paprika and Parmesan cheese. Place cut half down on oiled cookie sheet. Bake at 350° for 25 to 30 minutes until potato is fork tender.

Yield: 2 servings   Serving size: 1/2 potato

Per serving: Calories: 84
             Carbohydrate: 16 gms.
             Protein: 1 gm.
             Fat: 1 gm.
             Sodium: 38 mg.
             Exchanges: 1 starch/bread

Bulgur or cracked wheat is a tasty way to add fiber to your diet. The wheat has a mild, nutty flavor that goes well with all kinds of vegetables and meat, fish or poultry. It also has the advantage of cooking very quickly.

Vegetable Bulgur Pilaf*

1 small carrot, diced
1 medium stalk celery, diced
1/2 green pepper, diced
1/2 cup mushrooms, sliced
2 green onions, thinly sliced

1 bay leaf
1½ Tbsp. oil
3/4 cup vegetable stock or
   water
1 cup raw bulgur wheat
1/4 tsp. salt

Prepare the vegetables. Include some celery leaves (a few add a nice flavor; too many make the dish bitter). Place the oil in a heavy pot with a close-fitting lid. Add all the vegetables and the bay leaf. Stir over medium heat for several minutes. Pour in the stock, bring to a boil, cover and simmer for 5 minutes.

Add the wheat and salt and bring back to a fast boil. Cook, covered, over very low heat for 15 minutes. If too moist, uncover and simmer another few minutes until the liquid evaporates.

Yield: 4 servings

Serving size: 1/2 cup

Per serving: Calories: 217
Carbohydrate: 37 gms.
Fat: 6 gms.
Sodium: 292 mg.

Exchanges: 2 starch/bread
1 vegetable
1 fat

Syrup for Hot or Cold Chocolate Drink

1/2 cup unsweetened cocoa
Artificial sweetener equal to
   1/2 cup plus 2½ Tbsp. sugar

1/2 cup hot water
2 tsp. vanilla

In saucepan, combine cocoa, artificial sweetener, sugar, and water. Mix well. Cook over medium heat stirring constantly until mixture comes to boiling point. Stir in vanilla.

Store syrup in jar in refrigerator. Add 1 to 2 Tbsp., or less if desired, to skim milk allowance to make hot or cold chocolate. This cannot be used as a topping since it has a bitter taste before being mixed with milk.

Yield: 12 servings

Serving size: 2 Tbsp.

Per serving: Calories: 17
Carbohydrate: 2 gms.
Protein: 1 gm.

Fat: 5 gm.
Sodium: 262 mg.
Exchanges: free

Kool-Aid Mix

1 pkg. Kool-Aid (without sugar)
2¼-4 tsp. granulated artificial sweetener

Mix ingredients. Use 1/2 tsp. or more as desired of the mix per one cup of water. The mixture can be sealed in a plastic bag for travel or camping.

Yield: 8 cups   Serving size: 1 cup

Per serving: Calories: 4   Sodium: 1 mg.
               Carbohydrate: 1 gm.   Exchanges: free

Low Calorie Lemonade

Put 1/4 tsp. non-caloric liquid sweetener in 2 Tbsp. lemon juice. Add to 1 cup water. Add ice as desired.

Yield: 1 cup   Serving size: 1 cup

Per serving: Calories: 8   Sodium: trace
               Carbohydrate: 2 gms.   Exchanges: free

    The following recipes are from Camp Needlepoint (American Diabetes Association of Minnesota's camp for children with diabetes).

Homemade Granola

4 cups uncooked oatmeal (quick type)
1 cup chopped peanuts (no skins)
1/2 cup Grape Nuts
1/2 cup bran (unprocessed, uncooked)
Sugar substitute to equal 1/4 cup sugar
1/3 cup vegetable oil
1/2 cup wheat germ
1/2 cup raisins

Spread the oatmeal on a cookie sheet and heat in a 350° oven for 10 minutes. Combine all but the last two ingredients. Bake on an ungreased cookie sheet or pan for 20 minutes, stirring once to brown evenly. Allow mixture to cook in the oven. Add wheat germ and raisins. Refrigerate in glass jars or plastic containers. (Granulated sugar substitute was more acceptable than liquid sugar substitute in this product.)

Yield: 6½ cups (26 servings)   Serving size: 1/4 cup

Per serving: Calories: 140   Fat: 7 gms.
               Carbohydrate: 15 gms.   Sodium: 57 mg.
               Protein: 5 gms.   Exchanges: 1 starch/bread, 1 fat

Gorp

1 cup salted peanuts
1 cup raisins
1 cup sunflower seeds
1 cup of each cereal: bran, wheat, corn chex

Mix all the ingredients together for a tasty snack. Store in a air-tight container.

Yield: 6⅔ cups (20 servings)　　　　　　Serving size: 1/3 cup

Per serving:　Calories: 116　　　　Fat: 6 gms.
　　　　　　　Carbohydrate: 12 gms.　Sodium: 110 mg.
　　　　　　　Protein: 4 gms.　　　　Exchanges: 1 starch/bread
　　　　　　　　　　　　　　　　　　　　　　　　1 fat

Cocoa Mix

1/3 cup nonfat dry milk
2½ tsp. powdered unsweetened cocoa
2/3 tsp. granulated artificial sweetener

Mix ingredients thoroughly. For camping, seal in a plastic bag. Add 3/4 cup hot or cold water to dry mix, which is approximately 6 Tbsp.

Yield: 1 serving　　　　　　　　　　Serving size: 1 cup

Per serving:　Calories: 93　　　　Fat: trace
　　　　　　　Carbohydrate: 14 gms.　Sodium: 124 mg.
　　　　　　　Protein: 9 gms.　　　　Exchanges: 1 low fat milk

The smunchie recipes are from the Mason Clinic, Seattle, Washington, and are also served at Camp Needlepoint.

Banana Smunchies

2 cups peanut butter
2 cups ripe bananas, mashed
52 graham cracker squares

Mash very ripe bananas into a smooth paste. Mix in peanut butter. Chill well. Drop 2 Tbsp. onto one square graham cracker, cover with second graham cracker square. Freeze until ready to use.

Yield: 26 servings　　　　　　　Serving size: 1 smunchie

Per serving:　Calories: 188　　　　Fat: 11 gms.
　　　　　　　Carbohydrate: 20 gms.　Sodium: 118 mg.
　　　　　　　Protein: 7 gms.　　　　Exchanges: 1 starch/bread
　　　　　　　　　　　　　　　　　　　　　　　　1 medium fat meat
　　　　　　　　　　　　　　　　　　　　　　　　1 fat

Chocolate Smunchies

1 pkg. sugar-free chocolate pudding mix
2 cups nonfat milk
3 cups peanut butter
70 graham cracker squares

Mix chocolate pudding according to directions on package using nonfat milk. Cool thoroughly. Mix peanut butter with pudding. Drop 1 Tbsp. onto 1 square graham cracker. Place low-calorie whipped topping on top of the pudding/peanut butter mixture, cover with second graham cracker square. Freeze until ready to use.

Yield: 35 servings   Serving size: 1 smunchie

Per serving: Calories: 200   Sodium: 142 mg.
              Carbohydrate: 17 gms.   Exchanges: 1 starch/bread
              Protein: 8 gms.   1 medium fat meat
              Fat: 12 gms.   1 fat

Sugar-Free Popsicles

1 pkg. sugar-free gelatin   2 cups boiling water
1 pkg. Kool-Aid   2 cups cold water
1 Tbsp. artificial sweetener

Combine ingredients and freeze in trays with sticks.

Yield: 1 ice cube tray   Serving size: 1 popsicle

Per serving: Calories: negligible
              Sodium: trace
              Exchanges: free

Banana Pop

1 banana
1 Tbsp. wheat germ

Peel and cut the banana in half crosswise. Slide popsicle stick into cut end of banana half, roll in wheat germ, stand in jar, place in freezer.

Yield: 2 pops   Serving size: 1 pop

Per serving: Calories: 60   Fat: 1 gm.
              Carbohydrate: 13 gms. Sodium: trace
              Protein: 2 gms.   Exchanges: 1 fruit

These recipes are for the holiday foods included in the menus in Chapter 28.

Cauliflower Supreme

1 large head cauliflower
1-1½ cups boiling water
2 cups seeded or seedless grapes
1/4 cup slivered toasted almonds
1 tsp. salt

Break off each floweret of the cauliflower, then slice lengthwise into slices 1/4″ thick. Simmer in boiling water in a covered skillet for 5 minutes or until tender. Drain. Fold in green grapes and almonds. Serve immediately.

Yield: 6 servings   Serving size: 1 cup

Per serving: Calories: 83   Sodium: 390 mg.
             Carbohydrate: 12 gms.   Exchanges: 1/2 fruit
             Protein: 2 gms.   1 vegetable
             Fat: 4 gms.   1 fat

Cranberry-Celery Salad

1 envelope sugar-free   1 cup coarsely
   gelatin (strawberry or cherry)   ground cranberries
1 cup boiling water   1 cup chopped celery
1 Tbsp. lemon juice   1/2 cup cold water

Add boiling water to gelatin. Stir until dissolved. Add cold water. Chill until partly set. Add lemon juice, chopped cranberries and celery. Pour into decorative mold. Chill until set. Serve on lettuce.

Yield: 6 servings   Serving size: 1/6 of the mold

Per serving: Calories: 20   Fat: trace
             Carbohydrate: 5 gms.   Sodium: 22 mg.
             Protein: trace   Exchanges: 1 serving = free
                                                 3 servings = 1 fruit

Pumpkin Pie

Chilled uncooked pastry shell
3 eggs
1 tsp. pumpkin pie spice
2 Tbsp. melted margarine
1½ cups cooked or canned pumpkin
1½ cups scalded skim milk
1 Tbsp. sugar substitute

Beat eggs and add, in order, spices, salt, sweetener, melted margarine, pumpkin and scalded milk. Pour into pastry shell and bake at 450° for 10 minutes. Turn oven to 325° and continue baking for 30 minutes.

Yield: 1 pie, 6 servings   Serving size: 1/6 of the pie

Per serving: Calories: 204   Sodium: 226 mg.
             Carbohydrate: 18 gms.   Exchanges: 1 starch/bread
             Protein: 7 gms.   1 vegetable
             Fat: 12 gms.   2 fat

Flaming Cherries Jubliee

1 can (16 oz.) water packed or juice packed dark cherries
2 tsp. cornstarch
1 tsp. sugar
1/2 tsp. artificial liquid sweetener
1/4 cup cherry brandy
red food coloring
1/4 cup Cherry Kirsch (to flame)

Drain cherries. Add water to cherry liquid to make 3/4 cup. In saucepan, combine cornstarch and sugar; blend in cherry liquid. Cook and stir until thickened. Add cherries, liquid sweetener, cherry brandy and a few drops food coloring. Serve hot.

To Flame: Slowly heat Cherry Kirsch in small saucepan for a few minutes. DO NOT BOIL. Light with match and pour over cherries. (Be sure cherry mixture is hot.)

Yield: 4 servings   Serving size: 3/4 cup

Per serving: Calories: 61   Sodium: 2 mg.
             Carbohydrate: 14 gms.   Exchanges: 1 fruit
             Protein: trace

The cherry sauce may also be used to garnish other desserts. Spoon sauce over 1/2 cup vanilla ice cream (1 starch/bread and 2 fat exchanges) or over 1½″ cube sponge cake (1 starch/bread exchange).

Wiggley Easter Shapes

1 envelope sugar-free gelatin

Prepare gelatin using fruit juice in place of half of the water called for. Do not add any water. Pour into a small rectangular pan and refrigerate until set. Use Easter cookie cutters and cut into Easter shapes.

Yield: 4 servings   Serving size: 1/2 cup

Per serving: Calories: 56   Sodium: 9 mg.
             Carbohydrate: 14 gms.   Exchanges: 1 fruit

Bunny Salad

Place crisp lettuce leaf on a plate. Place upside down on top of it 2 chilled unsweetened pear halves. Make 2 bunnies, using narrow end for the face.

Eyes: 4 cloves
Nose: 2 pimento
Ears: 4 blanched whole almonds
Tail: Cottage cheese formed into 2 balls

Yield: 2 bunnies   Serving size: 2 bunnies

Per serving: Calories: 56   Sodium: 1 mg.
             Carbohydrate: 14 gms.   Exchanges: 1 fruit

Carrot Orange Toss

2 oranges, diced   1 tsp. lemon juice
2 cups grated carrots   1/2 cup raisins
2 Tbsp. honey

Combine all ingredients. Chill. Serve on lettuce cups.

Yield: 8 servings   Serving size: 1/2 cup

Per serving: Calories: 88   Sodium: 31 mg.
             Carbohydrate: 21 gms.   Exchanges: 1 fruit
             Protein: 1 gm.   1 vegetable

Here are other ideas for Easter treats.

Easter Sparkle Dessert

1 envelope lemon flavored sugar-free gelatin

1 envelope lime flavored sugar-free gelatin

Prepare the gelatin using the directions on the envelope of each package. Pour each flavor separately into a pie pan and place in the refrigerator to gel. As soon as the gelatin is set, take a sharp knife and cut into 1/2″ cubes. Pile the cubes into a sherbet glass, alternating the lemon and lime. This dessert really sparkles!

Yield: two 9″ pie pans   Serving size: 1/2 cup

Per serving: Calories: 8   Sodium: 8 mg.
             Carbohydrate: 2 gms.   Exchanges: up to 1
                                                 cup: free

Marshmallow Crispies

1 Tbsp. vegetable oil
40 large (or 4 cups miniature) marshmallows
4 cups crisp rice cereal

Grease large saucepan with cooking oil. Add marshmallows and melt over low heat; watch carefully. Quickly stir in cereal; mix well. With buttered spoon, press into greased 8 × 8 × 2-inch pan. Cut into 25 squares.

Yield: 25 squares   Serving size: 1 square

Per serving: Calories: 60   Fat: trace
              Carbohydrate: 15 gms.   Sodium: 39 mg.
              Protein: trace   Exchanges: 1 fruit

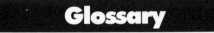

Beta cells: Specialized cells located in the islets of Langerhans of the pancreas. They manufacture insulin and release it into the bloodstream in response to food intake in order to keep blood glucose concentrations normal.

Blood glucose: Blood sugar. The principal fuel for most cells of the body. Normal fasting values are in the range of 70 to 120 milligrams per deciliter; with food intake, blood glucose levels will usually be under 140 to 160 milligrams per deciliter.

Calorie: A unit of measure used to express the energy value of food or the amount of energy used for activity. Nutrients supplying energy (calories) are carbohydrates, fat, protein and alcohol.

Carbohydrate: A nutrient in foods that is the major source of energy. Carbohydrates are sugars, starches and fiber.

> **Refined or simple carbohydrates:** Foods high in sugar content, such as soda pop, jam, jelly, honey, syrup, molasses, etc. They are a concentrated form of carbohydrate.

> **Complex or unrefined carbohydrates:** Foods primarily containing starch and often fiber, such as vegetables, breads, cereals, starchy vegetables, legumes, etc. They are usually not as concentrated a sweet as the refined carbohydrates.

CHO: Abbreviation for carbohydrate.

Counter-regulatory hormones: Often called "stress hormones," they are hormones that oppose the action of insulin. They raise blood glucose by breaking down glycogen, body fats and proteins. These hormones include glucagon, glucocorticoids, catecholamines and growth hormone.

Euglycemia: The state of having blood glucose levels within the normal range.

Fat: The nutrient in foods that provides the most concentrated source of calories. There are three basic types of fat — saturated, polyunsaturated and monounsaturated. Fats may be either animal or vegetable in origin and solid or liquid. Fats may also be visible or invisible in foods.

> **Saturated fat:** Usually a fat of animal origin, such as lard, butter or from meat products, characterized by being solid at room temperature.

> This includes fats found in meat and butterfat present in dairy products, such as whole milk, 2% milk, cheese, butter, ice cream, whipped and sour cream. Solid (hydrogenated)

vegetable shortenings and coconut and palm kernel oil are vegetable oils that are saturated. Cocoa butter in chocolate is another saturated fat. Excessive intake of these fats has been associated with high blood cholesterol levels.

Polyunsaturated fat: Primarily a fat of vegetable origin that is liquid at room temperature. These fats help reduce blood cholesterol although it is not understood how this happens. Safflower, corn, sunflower, soybean and cottonseed oils are polyunsaturated fats.

Monounsaturated fat: Previously believed to be a neutral fat that neither raised nor lowered blood cholesterol levels. More recent research has suggested that it decreases blood cholesterol levels, without lowering HDL (the "good") cholesterol. Examples include olive oil, peanut oil, olives, peanuts, and most other nuts (except walnuts, which are polyunsaturated).

Omega-3 fatty acids: A type of oil found most commonly in fish. It lowers triglycerides and cholesterol as well as decreasing the clotting of blood platelets. Fish oils are found in cold water and "fatty" fish such as salmon, tuna, mackerel, herring, trout, crab, shrimp, lobster, and cod.

Fiber: That portion of food that cannot be digested by the human digestive system. Usually these are the structural parts of plants, such as skins, stems and seeds. Found in fruits, vegetables, whole grain breads and cereals.

Glucagon: A hormone produced by the alpha cells of the pancreas. It opposes the action of insulin by signaling the liver to break down stored fuels (mainly glycogen), which causes blood sugar to rise.

Glucose: The simple sugar used by the body cells for energy. See "Blood glucose."

Gluconeogenesis: The process by which amino acids are converted to glucose in the liver.

Glycogen: The stored form of carbohydrate, stored in liver and muscles as a reserve source of fuel. During fasting or during an insulin reaction, glycogen is broken down to glucose and released into the bloodstream.

Glycosylated hemoglobin: Hemoglobin to which molecules of glucose have been irreversibly attached. Blood glucose levels are higher in poorly controlled diabetes, causing more hemoglobin to be glycosylated. The amount of glycosylated hemoglobin present at any given time reflects the average blood glucose level over the prior three to six weeks (the life of a mature red blood cell). It is used as a measure of overall blood glucose control.

Hormones: Chemical messengers that are released into the bloodstream and regulate a variety of processes at various locations in the body, which may be quite distant from the source of the hormone. Insulin is an example of a hormone.

Hydrogenation: The chemical process of adding hydrogen to a fat; this changes liquid vegetable oils (unsaturated fats) to solid or hydrogenated fat (saturated fat), such as solid vegetable shortenings.

> **Partially hydrogenated** means hydrogen atoms have been added to some (not all) of the carbon atoms. Hydrogenated fats may also be called **hardened fats.**

Hyperglycemia: High blood sugar. Elevation of blood glucose above the normal range for a given age and state of feeding. Too high a blood sugar level can lead to ketoacidosis.

Hypoglycemia: Low blood sugar. Levels of blood glucose below the normal range (80 mg./dl. or less). Too low a blood sugar can lead to an insulin "reaction" or insulin "shock."

IDDM: Insulin-dependent diabetes mellitus, also called Type I diabetes. Individuals with this form of diabetes are dependent on the administration of insulin for life. If not treated with insulin, they develop ketoacidosis.

Ketoacidosis: An acute metabolic state that can occur in diabetes when blood levels of insulin are inadequate, causing high blood sugar levels and ketones. Toxic ketonic acids accumulate in the blood, and ketones appear in the urine. If untreated, it can result in coma and death.

Ketone: A substance formed when the body uses body fat for energy.

> **Lipids:** General term for fats. Several different types of lipids circulate in the blood; two of major concern are cholesterol and triglycerides.

> **Cholesterol:** A fat-like waxy substance manufactured by the body; present only in foods of animal origin (liver, egg yolk, cheese, meats, high fat dairy products). Cholesterol does not supply energy but is necessary for many of the body's chemical processes. For example, it is necessary for cell membranes and is the starting substance for sex hormones, vitamin D and bile acids in the body. Too much cholesterol has been associated with the development of heart and blood vessel disease.

> **Triglycerides:** The primary form of fat found in food and also the way fat is transported in the bloodstream. They are also manufactured by the body to store extra calories as an energy source. When fat intake is excessive and when diabetes is poorly controlled, blood levels of triglycerides tend to be elevated.

Lipoproteins: Fat-protein complexes. Since fats do not dissolve in water (or blood), they are transported in the blood by proteins that are water soluble.

> **Very low density lipoproteins (VLDL):** The lipoprotein complex that primarily transports triglycerides.

> **Low density lipoproteins (LDL):** The lipoprotein complex that primarily transports cholesterol.

> **High density lipoproteins (HDL):** The "good" cholesterol; high levels appear to be protective against coronary heart disease. They are not affected by diet but rather by the exercise level of the individual.

NIDDM: Non-insulin-dependent diabetes mellitus, also called Type II diabetes. Individuals with this form of diabetes can frequently manage their condition by diet alone or by diet and oral agents. Some individuals may require insulin to keep blood glucose normal, but they are not ketosis-prone. Onset of NIDDM is usually after age 40.

Postprandial: After eating, usually between 1 to 2 hours.

Preprandial: Before eating.

Protein: A nutrient that is an indispensable constituent of every living cell — the "building block" of the body. Protein can also be used by the body as a secondary source of energy. Proteins are links of many smaller molecules called amino acids. Food sources of protein are both plant and animal.

> **Amino acids:** Building blocks of protein. There are 22 amino acids from which all proteins in nature, animal and plant, are made. The body can manufacture nonessential amino acids from carbohydrates and nitrogen. Nine of the amino acids cannot be manufactured by the body and must be received from food. These are called essential amino acids.

> **Animal protein:** Protein derived from animal sources such as eggs, milk, meat, fish and poultry. Animal proteins contain all the essential amino acids.

> **Vegetable protein:** Protein derived from plant sources, such as soybeans; peanuts; lentils; mung beans; dried black-eyed peas; red, white, pinto, black, garbanzo and lima beans; pumpkin, sunflower and sesame seeds; oatmeal; wheat germ; and whole wheat. Vegetable proteins are usually lacking in one or more of the essential amino acids, and so must be eaten in combination with other protein sources in order to form complete proteins.

P/S ratio: The ratio obtained by dividing the number of grams of polyunsaturated fat by the number of grams of saturated fat in a food. The higher the P/S ratio, the more polyunsaturated fat in the food. A P/S ratio greater than 1.5:1 is recommended.

Salt: Sodium chloride; compound of approximately 40 percent sodium.

> **Sodium:** A naturally occurring mineral found in a great variety of foods. The largest source of sodium in the diet is salt. High levels of sodium may cause high blood pressure to develop in people who have a predisposition (tendency) to this disorder.

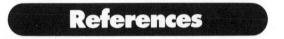

References

U.S. Department of Agriculture, U.S. Department of Health and Human Services: Nutrition and Your Health. Dietary Guidelines for Americans, Second Edition. Hyattsville, MD: U.S. Department of Agriculture, 1985.

American Diabetes Association Task Force on Nutrition and Exchange Lists: Nutritional recommendations and principles for individuals with diabetes mellitus: 1986. Diabetes Care 10(1): 126-132, 1987.

Franz M., Krosnick A., Maschak-Carey B.J., Parker T., Wheeler F.: Goals for Diabetes Education. Alexandria, VA: American Diabetes Association, 1986.

Franz M.J., Barr P., Holler H., Powers M.A., Wheeler M.L., Wylie-Rosett J: Exchange lists: Revised 1986. J Am Diet Assoc 87(1): 28-36, 1987.

American Diabetes Association, The American Dietetic Association: Exchange Lists for Meal Planning. Alexandria, VA: American Diabetes Association, 1986.

Etzwiler, D.D., Franz, M.J., Hollander, P., Joynes J: Learning to Live Well With Diabetes. Minneapolis, MN: Diabetes Centers, Inc. 1987.

Part I:

U.S.D.A. Agriculture Handbooks No. 8-1 to 14, 1976 to 1986.,

Pennington, J.A.T., and Church, H.N.: Bowes and Church's Food Values of Portions Commonly Used. 14th ed. Philadelphia, PA: J. B. Lippincott Co., 1985.

Kratzer, B.L., Sandt, D.W.: Nutrition: Where Have All These Labels Been? Phoenix, AZ: The Dallas Sandt Co. 1986.

Byerly's: Special Foods Shopping Guide for Expanded Food Exchanges. Minneapolis, MN: Byerly's, 1986.

The Buying Guide for Fresh Fruits, Vegetables, Herbs and Nuts. 7th ed. Hagerstown, MD: Blue Goose, Inc., 1980.

Franz, M.J., Hedding, B.K., Leitch, G.: Opening the Door to Good Nutrition. Minneapolis, MN: Diabetes Centers, Inc., 1985.

Monk, A., Franz, M. J.: Convenience Food Facts. Minneapolis, MN: Diabetes Centers, Inc., 1987.

Part II.

Anderson, J.W.: Plant Fiber in Foods. Lexington, KY: HCF Diabetes Research Foundation, Inc. 1986.

Wheeler, M.L., ed: Diabetes Mellitus and Glycemic Response to Different Foods: A Summary and Annotated Bibliography. Chicago, IL: Diabetes Care and Education Practice Group. American Diabetes Association, 1983, 1985.

American Diabetes Association, Washington, D.C. Affiliate, Inc: Supplement to Exchange Lists for Meal Planning Vegetarian Cookery; Oriental Cookery; Jewish. Bethesda, MD: Washington, D.C., Area Affiliate, Inc.

Truesdell, D.D., Whitney, E.N., Acosta, P.B: Nutrients in vegetarian foods. J.Am. Diet. Assoc. 84(1): 30-32, 1984.

Canadian Diabetes Association: Diabetes and Chinese Foods. Toronto, Ontario: Canadian Diabetes Association, 1978.

Hall, T.A., Bertram, K., Foerster, S.B.: Comer Bien para vivir mejor. A Professional Guide. Sacramento, CA: California Diabetes Control Program, 1985.

La Dieta Diabetica. Los Angeles, CA: Los Angeles District of the California Dietetic Association, 1977.

Planificacion de Comidas para Personas con Diabetes. Austin, TX: American Diabetes Association, Texas Affiliate, 1985.

Caribbean Food and Nutrrition Institute. Meal Planning for Diabetics. Kingston, Jamaica: Pan American Health Organizatgion, 1980.

Gleason, C.J., Jaquez, J.: Handbook of Mexican American Foods. San Antonio, TX: Intercultural Development Research Association, 1982.

Valley Baptist Medical Center Food Service Department: Descriptions of MexicanAmerican Foods and Nasco's Italian Foods. Fort Atkinson, WI: Nasco, 1979 and 1982.

Kahn, A.P.: Diabetes Control and the Kosher Diet. Skokie, IL: Wordscope Assoc., 1984.

Forgey, W.W.: The Complete Guide to Trail Food Use. 2nd ed. Pittsboro, IN: Indiana Camp Supply, Inc. 1977.

Part III.

Dining out with a healthy appetite. FDA Consumer. March: 19-23, 1987.

Franz, M.J.: Fast Food Facts. Minneapolis, MN. Diabetes Centers, Inc., 1987.

Franz, M.J.: Diabetes Mellitus: Considerations in the development of guidelines for the occasional use of alcohol. J. Am. Diet. Assoc. 83: 147-l51, 1983.

Franz, M.J.: Diabetes and Alcohol. Minneapolis, MN: Diabetes Centers, Inc. 1983.

Franz, M.J., Joynes, J.O.: Diabetes and Brief Illness. Minneapolis, MN: Diabetes Centers, Inc. 1987.

Franz, M.J.: Exercise and the management of diabetes. J. Am. Diet. Assoc. 87(7): 860-875, 1987.

Franz, M.J.: Exercise and diabetes mellitus in ed. Powers, M.: Handbook of Diabetes and Nutrition Management. Rockville, MD.: Aspen Systems Corporation, 1987.

Kris-Etherton, P.M.: Nutrition and the exercising female. Nutrition Today 21(2): 8, 1986.

Part IV.

Monk, A., Franz, M.J.: Convenience Food Facts. Minneapolis, MN: Diabetes Centers, Inc. 1987.

Cooper, N.: The Joy of Snacks. Minneapolis, MN: Diabetes Centers, Inc. 1987.

Franz, M.J.: Is it safe to consume aspartame during pregnancy? A review. Diabetes Educator. 12:145-147, 1986.

Crapo, P.: The use of alternative sweeteners in the diabetic diet. Diabetes Care, 1987.

MacRae, N.M.: Canning and Preserving Without Sugar. Seattle, WA: Pacific Search Press, 1982.

Franz, M.J., Hedding, B.K., Holtmeier, K., Monk, A., Siemers, D: A Guide to Healthy Eating. Minneapolis, MN: Diabetes Centers, Inc., 1985.

Franz, M.J., Hedding, B.K., Leitch, G.: Opening the Door to Good Nutrition. Minneapolis, MN: Diabetes Centers, Inc., 1985.

Franz, M.J., Hedding, B.K., Leitch, G.: Cooking to Stay in SHAPE. Minneapolis, MN: SHAPE, Park Nicollet Medical Foundation. 1981.

Index

Abalone, 81
Acidosis, 136, 152
Acree (Jamaican), 90
Aerobic dancing, 150
Alba 66 and 77, 42, 193
Alcohol, 1, 8, 130-133; exchanges for,
    134; guidelines for, 131-133; and
    hypoglycemia, 130-131; and
    metabolism, 130
Alcoholic beverages, composition of, 133;
    exchanges for, 134
Ale, 133
Alfalfa, 33, 77
Alfredo sauce, 98
All Bran, 67
Allen, Dr. Frank, 22
Almond cookies, 83
Almonds, 46, 75; recipe exchange, 214
Amaramthus, 90
American Cancer Society, 5, 64
American cheese spread, 23
American Diabetes Association, 4, 5, 196
American Dietetic Association, 3, 10
American Heart Association, 5
American Pasteurized Process cheese, 27
Amino acid; defined, 235; need for 72-73
Anchiote, 46
Anchovies, 82; fillets, 24
Angel food cake, 56
Animal cookies, 56
Animal crackers, 16, 191
Animal protein. *See also* Protein. defined,
    235
A-1 Sauce, 48
Appendicitis, 64
Appetizers, 120
Apple(s), 64; baked, 56; banana, 90;
    Brown Betty, 56; cider, 193;
    crabapple, 36
Apricot(s), dried, salted, 83; nectar, 37
Arabic bread, 74
Arby's, 127-128
Arrowroot, 82; starch, 81
Arroz con pollo, 92-93
Artichoke, 31-33
Asparagus, 32
Aspartame, 7, 196-199
Atherosclerosis, 2
Au gratin potatoes, 14
Autopsy, 2
Avocado, 45, 90

Baby Swiss cheese, 23
Backpacking. *See* Camping
Bacon; bacon, lettuce, tomato sandwich,
    53; exchanges, 28, 44; recipe
    exchange, 220; substitute, 74
Badminton, 150
Bagel, 102; defined, 104
Baked bean with bacon soup, 17
Baking, 44
Bamboo shoots, 32, 77, 82
Banana; bread, 15; pop, recipe for, 228;
    Smunchies, recipe for, 227
Barbecue; ribs, 25, 28; sauce, recipe for,
    213
Barley, 13, 68, 74, 204
Basketball; calories required, 150; and
    food adjustment, 144
Bean(s); baked, 69; with bacon soup, 17;
    with franks, 112; black, 74; cooking
    time, 299; dried, 69, 207; frijoles, 89;
    and ham, 51; horse, 81; Mexican, 89,
    94; red mung, 81; refired, 89;
    Romano, 98-99; tofu, 25; yard-long,
    33; yellow snap, 32
Bean sprouts, 77, 82, 85
Beef, 20-21, 23, 25-26; blood sausage, 27;
    blade steak, 23; chili soup, 17; dried
    chipped, 111; jerky, 20, 111, 192;
    noodle soup, 17; recipe exchange,
    215; roast, Arby's, Rax, 127-128; stew,
    112; stroganoff, 112; tongue, 102; and
    vegetables, 84; vegetable stew, 51
Beer, 133-134
Beets, cooked, 32
Beta cells, 232
Beverages, convenience, 187; malt, non
    alcoholic, 133-134. *See also*
    Carbonated beverages; Milk; Soda
Bialy, 102
Bicycling; calories for, 150; and food
    adjustment, 144
Big Franks, 76
Bile salts, 64
Biscuit(s), 110; breakfast, 125; fast food,
    125; mix exchange, 210
Bitter melon, 82, 85
Black Diamond cheese, 26
Blackeyed peas, 14
Blade steak, beef, 23
Blood sausage, 27
Blintzes, cheese, 104
Blood cholesterol. *See* Cholesterol
Blood fat. *See* Saturated fat; Unsaturated
    fat.
Blood glucose, 2, 4, 6, 8, 55-56; defined,
    232; and exercise, 139; and illness,
    135-138; monitoring, 8; and snacking,
    188-193

238

Gas, and fiber, 65-66
Gastrointestinal problems, 64
Gatorade, 38
Gazpacho, 90, 98
Gefilte fish, 103, 105
Gelatin, 49, 59; dessert, 58; pops, 193
Ghee, 90
Ginger, 82; bread, 56, 112; snaps, 192
Ginkgo seeds, 81, 86
Glucagon, defined, 233
Glycogen, defined, 233
Gluconeogenesis, defined, 233
Glucose, 195. See also Blood glucose;
    defined, 233
glycoslated hemogloben, defined, 233
Glutinous flour, 81
Glutinous rice, 81; defined, 86
Glycemic control, 65; and alcohol, 130-
    131
Goat's milk, 42, 77
Goldfish crackers, 16
Golfing; calorie requirement, 150; food
    adjustment for, 144
Good cholesterol. See Lipoprotein
Gooseberries, 36
Goose liver pate, 46
Gorp, 110; recipe for, 226
Gort, 89
Gouda cheese, 27
Gow-Gee, 84
Graham crackers, 68, 110; crumb, recipe
    exchange, 210
Granadillo, 37-38
Granola, 12, 110; bar, 58, 110; recipe for,
    225
Grapefruit, 37
Gravy, 47; Weight Watchers, 50
Grebnes, 104
Green beans, 111
Green River skim milk cheese, 24
Griddle steaks (vegetarian), 77
Grilled cheese sandwish, 53
Grits, 68
Groats, 13, 74, 102, 205
Ground beef, 21
Gruyere, 27
Guacamole, 90, 94
Guava, 37, 83, 90, 94; nectar, 90
Gumdrops, 59

Ham, 22, 111; country style, 28; and lima
    bean casserole, 52; sandwich, 53
Hamburger, 25; deluxe, fastfood, 125;
    exchange list, 126-127
Hamburger Helper, 186
Hard Roll, 15
Hardee's, 127

Har-Gow, 84
Hashed brown potatoes, 14, 110
Hawaiian Punch, 38, 193
HDL. See Lipoprotein, high-density
Head cheese, 27
Heart disease, 2-3, 5, 7, 64-65; and fiber,
    65
Hemicelluloses, 63
Hemorrhoids and fiber, 64
Herring, pickled (kippered), 24, 103
Hickory Smoked cheese, 26
High fat diet, 2
High blood pressure. See Blood pressure
Hi Ho crackers, 16, 191
Hoagie, 54
Hockey; calorie requirements, 150; food
    adjustments for, 144
Holiday menus, 169-172
Hominy, 13, 89
Homli fruit, 37, 38
Hommous, 77 75 78
Honey, 49, 195; recipe exchange, 214
Honey Nut Cheerios, 12
Hoop cheese, 21
Hormones, counter-regulatory, 232
Hops (bread), 89
Hors d'oeuvres, 170. See also Snacks
Horse beans, 81
Horseradish, 49
Hotdish. See Casserole; combination
    foods
Hotdog, 54; with cheese, 125; with chili,
    127; fast food exchange, 127
Hot 'N Spicy, 26
Hush puppies, 110
Hydrogenated vegetable oil, 47
Hyperglycemia, 140-141
Hypertension, 65
Hypoglycemia, 8, 65; and alcohol, 130-
    132; and exercise, 140; and snacking,
    188-193

Ice cream, 6, 10; bars, 57; cone, 58, 125.
    See also Comet cone; milk, 57;
    sandwich, 57
Identification; and exercise, 143; for
    traveling, 152
Illness; and diabetic control, 135-138;
    and traveling, 156-161
Imitation ingredients, 177
Ingredient listing on labels, 178
Interchanges, 118-119
Invert sugar, 95
Insulin; dependence on 5-6, 8; and diet,
    5-6, 8; discovery of, 1-2; and eating
    out, 118-119; and exercise, 141-146;
    and fiber, 65; and holiday eating, 169-

172; and illness, 135-138; and snacking, 188-192; and traveling, 152-161; Italian cooking, 97-100

Jalapeno beans, 49, 90
Jam, 49
Japanese cooking. *See* Oriental cooking
Jarlsberg, 27
Java plum cheese, 37
Jell-O, recipe exchange, 214
Jelly, 49
Jelly beans, 59
Jewish cooking, 101-107
Jicama, 32, 34, 89-90, 94
Jogging; caloric requirement, 150; and food adjustment, 144
The Joy of Snacks (Cooper), 189
Juan canary melon, 40
Juice, fruit. *See also* specific fruit list of 37-38
Jumping rope, 150
Junk foods, legal, 191-193

Kabob cubes, 21
Kaiser roll, 15, 103
Kale, 32
Kasha, 13, 68, 74, 78, 102, 105, 207
Kashruth, 101
Kavli, 192
Kefir, 77-78
Kentucky Fried Chicken, Original recipe, 128
Ketones, in illness, 136-137
Kichel, 103
Kidney beans, 75
Kidney disease, 7
Kippered herring, 103
Kiwi fruit, 37-39
Knish, potato, 103, 105
Knockkwurst, 27
Kohlrabi, 32, 34, 82
Kool-Aid, 49; recipe for, 225
Korean cooking. *See* Oriental cooking
Kosher, defined, 101
Kreplach, meat, 104-105
Kugel, potato, 103-105
Kumquat, 37-39, 83, 86

Label reading, 175-183; ingredients, 178; nutrition, 178-181; terms, 176-178
Lacto-ovo-vegetarian, sample menu, 78-79
Lactose, 195
Lady finger cookie, 57
Lamb, 22, 25
Lard substitution, 219
Lasagna, 99-100, 113
Latke, 103, 106

Laughing Cow cheese, 21
Lean meat, list of, 20-23
Lean 'n Tasty, 26
Lecithin, 77
Leek, 32, 34, 82
Legumes, 78, 205, 207; as fiber, 66; in vegetarian diet, 73
Lemon, 37; -ade, recipe for, 225; drops, 59; juice, 38; rind, 49
Lentils, 75; as fiber, 66
Lifesavers, 59
Lifestyle, 5
Light foods, 177, 185
Light 'n Lively American Cheese, 21
Lignin, 63
Lima beans, 69
Lime, 37; juice, 38
Lipid levels, 65
Lipoprotein, high-density, 65; defined, 235; high density (HDL), 235; low density (LDL), 235; very low density (VLDL), 235
Liqueurs, 133, 134
Lite-Line, 21
Liver, chopped, 103-104
Liverwurst, 27, 54
Lobster, 22; Maine, Red Lobster, 129
Loganberries, 36
London broil, 21
Longhorn Lyte, 26
Loquats, 37-39, 86
Lorna Doone shortbread, 57
Lorraine Swiss, 26
Lotus; root, 82, 86; seeds, 82
Low blood sugar. *See* Hypoglycemia
Lowfat milk. *See* Milk
Lox (smoked salmon), 103, 106
Lukshen, 103
Luncheon meats, 27-28, 44
Lychee nuts (litchis), 37, 39, 83, 86

Macademia nuts, 46
Macaroni, recipe exchange, 211
Macaroni and cheese, 113, 186
Mackeral, 24
Malanga, 13, 19, 89, 94
Malt-O-Meal, 12
Malt powder, 58
Maltose, 195
Mamey, 90
Mango, 39, 90
Manicotti, 99-100
Mannose, 195
Mannitol, 195
Maple syrup, 59, 112, 195; recipe for, 223
Margerine, 45, 112; recipe exchange, 212

Ovaltine, 49
Ox tail, 82
Oyster plant, 14
Oyster(s); breaded, 24; fried, 24; raw, 22;
    stew, 18

Palm oil, 29, 47
Pancakes, 16, 110; potato, 52
Pan spray, vegetable, 50
Papaya, 90
Parmesan cheese, 24; recipe exchange,
    212
Parsnips, 14
Pasta, 66, 98, 100
Pastrami, 27
Pastry, 58
Patty shell, 15, 58
Pea(s); black-eyed, 75; cow, 75; garden,
    69; pods, 32; split, 75
Peach nectar, 38
Peanut butter, 28, 54, 76, 111; recipe
    exchange, 214
Peanuts, 28, 111; recipe exchange, 214;
    roasted, 76
Pear nectar, 38
Pecans, 46, 76; recipe exchange, 214
Pectin, 63
Pepperidge Farm Goldfish, 191
Pepperoni, 27
Pepper steak, 85
Persian melon, 40
Persimmon, 39
Phenylketonuria (PKU), 197
Philadelphia Light cheese, 24
Physical activity. See Exercising
Picadillo, 92
Pickle(s); dill, 49; relish, 49
Pickled herring, 103
Pie crust, 58; meat, 186
Pignolias, 28, 46, 76
Pig's feet, 28
Pimento, 32, 49; cheese, 27
Pineapple, 37
Pinenuts, 28, 46, 76
Pinto beans, 75
Pistachio nuts, 28, 46, 76
Pizza, 10, 99, 128; with cheese, 52;
    frozen, 186; plain, 52
Plantains, 37-39, 69, 89, 94
Pocket bread, 15
Poi, 81
Poiret fruit spread, 37
Polaner all fruit, 37
Pollo alla tetrazzini, 98
Polish sausage, 27
Polyunsaturated fat, 44; defined, 233
Pomegranate, 39

Popcorn, 68, 191, 205; microwave, 17
Popover, 15
Popsicle, 58; sugar free, recipe, 227
Pork; belly, fresh, 28; chops, 111; feet, 82;
    hock, smoked, 28; roast, 23; roast and
    gravy, 54
Port du Salut, 27
Porterhouse steak, 23
Postprandial, defined, 235
Postum, 49
Pot cheese, 21, 103
Potatoe, 14, 103; au gratin, 14, 186;
    baked, 69, 128; chips, 17, 191; diced,
    110; as fiber, 66; flakes, 14;
    hashbrowns, 14, 110; mashed, 118;
    quick baked, recipe, 223; stuffed, 124;
    pancake, 52; puffs, 14; salad, 53;
    scalloped, 14; shoestring, 14; soup,
    cream of, 18; sweet, 14, 69
Poultry, 22-23, 25
Poundcake, 56
Preprandial, defined, 235
Preserving food. See Canning; Freezing
Pretzels, 17, 191
Prickley pears, 37, 39
Prime beef, 25
Prosciutto, 98
Protein, 1, 2, 7, 9, 23, 29, 41; animal,
    defined, 235
Provolone, 27, 98
Prunes, 111
P/S ratio, defined, 235
Pudding(s), 58, 112, 193; pop, 58, 192
Puffed; corn, 13; rice, 13; wheat, 13
Pumpkin, 33; bread, 16; seeds, 28, 46, 76

Quesadillas, 92, 95
Queso fresco, 89, 95; Mexican, 89;
    Jalisco, 89
Quick bread mixes, 186
Quince, 37, 39

Rabbit, 22
Raisin(s), 112, 193; recipe exchange,
    213
Raisin Bran, 12
Ralston, whole wheat, 68
Ramaki, 85
Racquetball; caloric requirement, 151;
    and food adjustment, 144
Raspberries, 37
Ratatouille, 98
Ravioli, 99, 100
Rax, 127-128
Rax, Ham 'n Cheese, 128
Recipe exchanges, 210-216
Recipe modification, 218-221

If you found this book helpful and would like more information on this and other related subjects you may be interested in one or more of the following titles from our *Wellness and Nutrition Library.*

BOOKS:

The Joy of Snacks — Good Nutrition for People Who Like to Snack
(288 pages)
The Physician Within (210 pages)
Pass The Pepper Please (90 pages)
Fast Food Facts (40 pages)
Convenience Food Facts (137 pages)
Opening The Door To Good Nutrition (186 pages)
Learning To Live Well With Diabetes (392 pages)
Exchanges For All Occasions (210 pages)
A Guide To Healthy Eating (60 pages)

BOOKLETS & PAMPHLETS

Diabetes & Alcohol (4 pages)
Diabetes & Exercise (20 pages)
Emotional Adjustment To Diabetes (16 pages)
Healthy Footsteps For People With Diabetes (13 pages)
Diabetes Record Book (68 pages)
Diabetes & Brief Illness (8 pages)
Diabetes & Impotence: A Concern for Couples (6 pages)
Adding Fiber To Your Diet (10 pages)
Gestational Diabetes: Guidelines for A Safe Pregnancy and Healthy Baby
(24 pages)
Recognizing and Treating Insulin Reactions (4 pages)
Hypoglycemia (functional) (4 pages)

The *Wellness and Nutrition Library* is published by Diabetes Center, Inc. in Minneapolis, Minnesota, publishers of quality educational materials dealing with health, wellness, nutrition, diabetes and other chronic illnesses. All our books and materials are available nationwide and in Canada through leading bookstores. If you are unable to find our books at your favorite bookstore contact us directly for a free catalog:

Diabetes Center, Inc.
P.O. Box 739
Wayzata, MN 55391